Diabetes and Cardiovascular Disease

W0043337

Francesco Paneni
Francesco Cosentino

Diabetes and Cardiovascular Disease

A Guide to Clinical Management

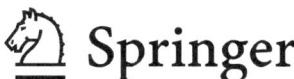 Springer

Francesco Paneni
Cardiology Unit
Karolinska University
Hospital
Solna
Stockholm
Sweden

Francesco Cosentino
Cardiology Unit
Karolinska University
Hospital
Solna
Stockholm
Sweden

ISBN 978-3-319-17761-8   ISBN 978-3-319-17762-5   (eBook)
DOI 10.1007/978-3-319-17762-5

Library of Congress Control Number: 2015942672

Springer Cham Heidelberg New York Dordrecht London

Printed on acid-free paper

Springer International Publishing AG Switzerland is part of Springer Science+Business Media (www.springer.com)

Foreword

In the current environment, cardiovascular disease continues to be one of the causes – if not the leading cause – of mortality worldwide. Therefore, it is important to have publications and books, which provide appropriate perspective on the clinical management of these conditions. What makes this book timely and clinically relevant is linking it to the ongoing worldwide epidemic of diabetes, which appears to be a major factor for retarding the rate of decline in cardiovascular disease.

This book not only describes the various cardiovascular diseases and pathologies that are particularly predominant in the diabetic population, such as accelerated atherosclerosis, stroke, peripheral vascular disease and cardiomyopathy, but also addresses in a contemporary manner the major risk factors that lead to the increased burden of cardiovascular disorders in individuals with diabetes. Such risk factors include hypertension, thrombosis and dyslipidemia.

The pathogenesis of diabetes-related cardiovascular disorders has not been fully elucidated. The last decade of research has led to an explosion in our knowledge base in the field of diabetes and cardiovascular disease, due to the increasing use of state of the art techniques, including unbiased approaches such as next generation sequencing, increased interest in epigenetic approaches to explore gene/environment interactions, use of animal models to define, at a molecular and biochemical level, important pathways leading to disease, and sophisticated methods to measure lipids, proteins, DNA and RNA in various human samples. If this will lead to new treatments aimed at preventing or reducing the burden of disease, is still to be determined. However, this book provides a comprehensive and contemporary summary of the current treatments available. This includes anti-thrombotics, lipid lowering drugs, antihypertensive agents, and drugs specifically indicated for heart failure. There is a significant number of controversies in managing the diabetic patient and these are addressed in this book. This includes appropriate use of various anti-platelet agents and the optimal approach to address coronary artery disease in individuals with diabetes. A major issue relates to modern management of glycemic control in the diabetic population. With a dramatic increase in the number of medications available to lower glucose and the requirement by regulatory authorities to assess the impact of new glucose lowering agents on cardiovascular disease and mortality in diabetes, this topic remains an area of active clinical investigation. Furthermore, with the possibility that certain glucose lowering agents may be associated with effects in either increasing or reducing hospitalization for heart failure, the impact of glucose lowering drugs continues to be regularly monitored in the ongoing clinical trials.

Diabetic subjects, though in general at high risk of developing cardiovascular disease, are markedly different in terms of prognosis. It is hoped that identification of biomarkers or use of new vascular imaging approaches will help to identify those at highest risk who would be candidates for more aggressive multifactorial intervention to reduce cardiovascular burden and overt clinical disease. This book addresses the use of various available risk engines as well as providing a balanced summary of the current status of a range of putative biomarkers.

In summary, this practical yet scientifically rigorous book will interest not only clinicians but also researchers who want to learn more about cardiovascular disease in the diabetic population. Since diabetes is a common cause of premature cardiovascular disease, and cardiovascular disease, in turn, is responsible for more than 60 % of deaths in diabetic subjects, this book will interest cardiologists, endocrinologists (including diabetologists), general physicians and family doctors with a particular interest in diabetes.

With the increased knowledge, better understanding of the complexity of cardiovascular disease in the diabetic patient and improved treatment approaches, it is hoped that over the next decade we will see a further reduction in the burden of cardio-vascular disease, particularly in the setting of concomitant diabetes.

Mark Cooper
Baker IDI Heart and Diabetes Institute,
The Alfred Medical Research and Education Precinct
Melbourne, VIC, Australia

Contents

Part I
Diagnosis and Mechanisms
of Disease

Chapter 1
Epidemiology, Definition, and Diagnosis of Diabetes Mellitus

1.1 Global Burden of Diabetes

The prevalence of metabolic diseases such as obesity and diabetes (DM) is alarmingly increasing over the globe [1, 2]. The main determinants behind this process are represented by modifiable (environment, overnutrition, sedentary habits, smoking) and nonmodifiable factors such as genetic susceptibility and aging [3]. An important aspect to consider is that environmental changes have a strong legacy effect over the next generations [4–6]. In other words, long-term high caloric regimens and physical inactivity are capable to derail gene expression and cellular programs, and these alterations may be transmitted to the offspring thereby anticipating metabolic traits even in young, normoweight individuals [4, 7]. In line with this emerging notion, obesity and prediabetes are exploding in young adolescents and represent a major public health problem [1, 8]. Epidemiological analysis show that 6.9 % of the global population (316 million people) is currently affected by impaired glucose tolerance (IGT) and, most importantly, projections anticipate a dramatic IGT increase with more that 470 million people affected by the year 2035 (Fig. 1.1). Such

F. Paneni, F. Cosentino, *Diabetes and Cardiovascular Disease:*
A Guide to Clinical Management, DOI 10.1007/978-3-319-17762-5_1,
© Springer International Publishing Switzerland 2015

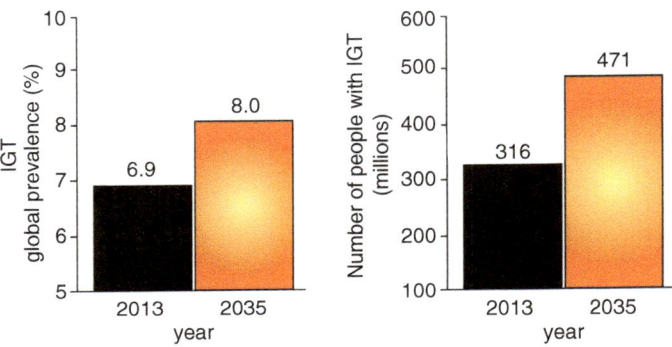

Fig 1.1 Worldwide prevalence of impaired glucose tolerance (Modified from International Diabetes Federation (IDF) [1]). *IGT* impaired glucose tolerance

pandemic of metabolic syndromes and obesity-related disorders hints a proportional increase in the prevalence of type 2 diabetes (T2D). The link between environmental factors, obesity, and subsequent dysglycemia indicates that the progression to DM occurs along a "continuum," not necessarily linear with time, which involves different cellular mechanisms including tissue-specific alterations of insulin signaling, changes in glucose transport, pancreatic beta cell dysfunction as well as deregulation of key genes involved in oxidative stress and inflammation [9–11]. Prevalence of metabolic disorders in adolescents is further boosted by pregnancy-related DM [12, 13]. Indeed, 21 million of live births were affected by DM only in the year 2013, suggesting that uterine environment plays a pivotal role (Table 1.1) [14].

Nowadays, 382 million people are affected by DM worldwide with most of cases registered in Western Pacific (138 million), South East Asia (72 million), and Europe (56 million) (Table 1.2) [1]. The majority of the 382 million people with DM are aged between 40 and 59, and 80 % of them

Table 1.1 Hyperglycemia in pregnancy in women (20–49 years)

Global prevalence (%)	16.9
Comparative prevalence (%)	14.8
Number of live births with hyperglycemia in pregnancy (millions)	21.4
Proportion of cases that may be due to diabetes in pregnancy (%)	16.0

Data from International Diabetes Federation (IDF) [1]

Table 1.2 Global forecasts of the number of people with diabetes from 2013 to 2035

Region	2013 (millions)	2035 (millions)	Increase %
Africa	19.8	41.4	109
Middle-East and North Africa	34.6	67.9	96
South-East Asia	72.1	123	71
South and Central America	24.1	38.5	60
Western Pacific	138.2	201.8	46
North America and Caribbean	36.7	50.4	37
Europe	56.3	68.9	22
World	**381.8**	**591.9**	**55**

Data from International Diabetes Federation (IDF) [1]

live in low- and middle-income countries. Most importantly, in these regions the disease remains largely undiagnosed (Table 1.3). Indeed almost 50 % of the people living in Western Pacific and South East Asia are not aware of the disease and remain undiagnosed for many years, leading to clear delays in the application of prevention and treatment strategies. Estimates by the International Diabetes Federation forecast that 592 million individuals will be affected by DM in 2035 (Table 1.2). This indicates that disease prevalence may increase by 55 % in only 22 years. Interestingly, new cases of DM will be mostly detected in Africa (109.1 %), Middle East and North Africa (96.2 %) as well

Table 1.3 Proportion of undiagnosed cases of diabetes in 2013 (20–79 years)

Region	Undiagnosed cases (%)
Africa	62
South-East Asia	49
South and Central America	24
Western Pacific	54
North America and Caribbean	27
Europe	48

Data from International Diabetes Federation (IDF) [1]

as South East Asia (70.6 %). By contrast, trajectories of DM prevalence are expected to be smoother in developed countries such as North America and Europe (Table 1.2). These differences might be explained by the fact that different forms of the disease are growing over the globe. Type 1 diabetes (T1D) is characterized by reduced pancreatic insulin secretion [15]. Several factors may contribute to T1D, including genetics and exposure to specific viruses triggering altered immune response and subsequent beta cell disruption (Fig. 1.2). Although T1D usually appears during childhood or adolescence, it also can begin in adults. In the latter condition, known as latent auto-immune DM in adults (LADA), insulin dependence develops over a few years.

T2D is a multifactorial disease, generally preceded by a state of overweight and characterized by the combination of insulin resistance (IR), increased free fatty acids (FFAs), and hyperglycemia (Fig. 1.2). Regardless of the underlining causes, DM represents a huge and growing problem with exponential costs for the society. This is particularly true for low-income countries where such DM epidemic will not be affordable by health care systems, with further increase of morbidity and mortality. DM is indeed one of the biggest killers together with cancer and cardiovascular disease, being responsible of 5.1 million death and USD 584 billion dollars expenditures only in the year 2013 [16].

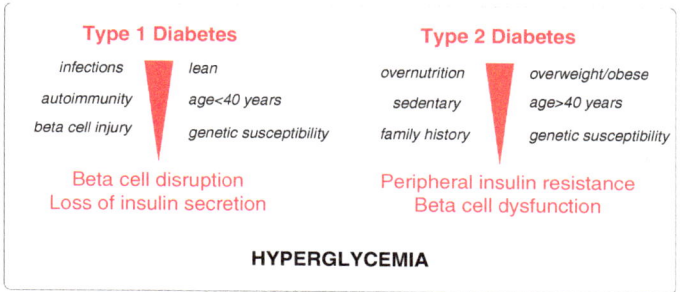

Fig. 1.2 Pathophysiology and risk factors associated with occurrence of type 1 and type 2 diabetes

1.2   Definition

DM is a complex disease characterized by an array of different mechanisms ultimately resulting in elevated blood glucose levels [17]. The disease is associated with high morbidity and mortality due to several complications occurring in multiple organs, including the cardiovascular system (coronary heart disease, peripheral artery disease, heart failure, and stroke). DM also affects the kidneys (diabetic nephropathy), the eyes (retinopathy), the peripheral nervous system (neuropathy), and the limbs (foot ulcers, amputations, Fig. 1.3). Beside these complications, DM increases susceptibility to infections, cancer, cognitive decline, and gastrointestinal disease. T1D is usually diagnosed in children and young adults, and was previously known as juvenile diabetes [18]. Only 5 % of people with DM have this form of the disease [16]. In contrast, patients who develop T2D are generally sedentary and obese. The progression from IGT to T2D may take many years to occur, leading to different intermediate disease phenotypes with continuous changes in glucose parameters and shifts in glucose tolerance category [3, 19]. Hence, understanding the

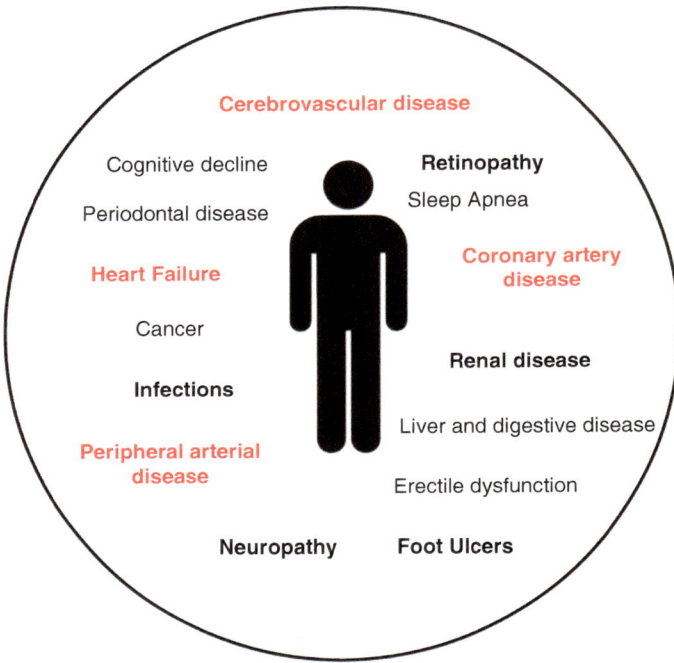

Fig. 1.3 Schematic representing diabetes-related comorbidities

factors predisposing to T2D is a major challenge. A growing form of DM is gestational diabetes which develops during pregnancy [20]. After delivery, most return to a euglycemic state, but they are at increased risk for overt T2D in the future. A meta-analysis reported that subsequent progression to DM is considerably increased after gestational DM. A large Canadian study found that the probability of DM developing after gestational DM was 4 % at 9 months and 19 % at 9 years after delivery [21].

Table 1.4 Cut-points for the diagnosis of impaired fasting glucose (IGF), impaired glucose tolerance (IGT), and diabetes

Condition	Criteria
Diabetes	
HbA$_{1c}$	≥6.5 % (48 mmol/mol)
FPG	≥7.0 mmol/L (≥126 mg/dL)
2hPG	≥11.1 mmol/L (≥200 mg/dL)
IGT	
FPG	<7.0 mmol/L (<126 mg/dL)
2hPG	7.8–11.0 mmol/L (140–198 mg/dL)
IFG	
FPG	5.6–6.9 mmol/L (100–125 mg/dL)
2hPG	<7.8 mmol/L (<140 mg/dL)

HbA1c glycated hemoglobin, *FPG* fasting plasma glucose, *IFG* impaired fasting glucose, *IGT* impaired glucose tolerance, *2hPG* 2-h plasma glucose

1.3   Diagnosis

In most of cases DM is a silent disease and half of the 382 million individuals with diabetes in 2013 were unaware of their diagnosis. Moreover, 300 million individuals show early features of altered glucose homeostasis, leading to a future risk of developing DM. Despite advances in diagnosis and treatment, we are still far from the identification of a reliable hyperglycemic marker for the detection of DM. DM is generally diagnosed when fasting plasma glucose (FPG) levels are ≥126 mg/dL in two different determinations (Table 1.4). Glycated hemoglobin (HbA$_{1c}$) has been recently introduced as a diagnostic test in combination with fasting plasma glucose (FPG). HbA$_{1c}$ is indeed a simple marker which may accurately reflect a condition of chronic hyperglycemia or altered glucose homeostasis [22]. However, there remain concerns regarding its sensitivity in predicting DM [23, 24]. According to new recommendations, an HbA_{1c} value ≥ 6.5 % together with FPG ≥ 126 mg/dL is sufficient to diagnose the disease. However, these two indices may be discordant and create uncertainties on whether DM is present or not. In these cases, an oral glucose tolerance test (OGTT) is highly recommended. This test is simple and reproducible and is able to unmask latent diabetes with high sensitivity and specificity [25]. OGTT values between 140 and 199 mg/dL identify a state of IGT, whereas values ≥ 200 mg/dL are compatible with DM. Therefore, OGTT may be required in the following conditions: (1) when FPG and HbA1c are discordant and (2) in all cases where IGT is suspected [26].

References

1. International Diabetes Federation (2013) IDF diabetes atlas, 6th edn. International Diabetes Federation, Brussels. http://www.idf.org/diabetesatlas
2. Hossain P, Kawar B, El Nahas M (2007) Obesity and diabetes in the developing world – a growing challenge. N Engl J Med 356:213–215
3. Paneni F, Costantino S, Cosentino F (2014) Insulin resistance, diabetes, and cardiovascular risk. Curr Atheroscler Rep 16:419
4. Napoli C, Crudele V, Soricelli A, Al-Omran M, Vitale N, Infante T et al (2012) Primary prevention of atherosclerosis: a clinical challenge for the reversal of epigenetic mechanisms? Circulation 125:2363–2373
5. Paneni F, Costantino S, Volpe M, Luscher TF, Cosentino F (2013) Epigenetic signatures and vascular risk in type 2 diabetes: a clinical perspective. Atherosclerosis 230:191–197
6. Barua S, Junaid MA (2015) Lifestyle, pregnancy and epigenetic effects. Epigenomics 7:85–102
7. Bouret S, Levin BE, Ozanne SE (2015) Gene-environment interactions controlling energy and glucose homeostasis and the developmental origins of obesity. Physiol Rev 95:47–82
8. Caprio S (2012) Development of type 2 diabetes mellitus in the obese adolescent: a growing challenge. Endocr Pract 18:791–795
9. Eckel RH, Kahn SE, Ferrannini E, Goldfine AB, Nathan DM, Schwartz MW et al (2011) Obesity and type 2 diabetes: what can be unified and

what needs to be individualized? J Clin Endocrinol Metab 96: 1654–1663

10. Paneni F, Beckman JA, Creager MA, Cosentino F (2013) Diabetes and vascular disease: pathophysiology, clinical consequences, and medical therapy: part I. Eur Heart J 34:2436–2443

11. Giacco F, Brownlee M (2010) Oxidative stress and diabetic complications. Circ Res 107:1058–1070

12. Jones RH, Ozanne SE (2007) Intra-uterine origins of type 2 diabetes. Arch Physiol Biochem 113:25–29

13. Cheung NW, Lih A, Lau SM, Park K, Padmanabhan S, McElduff A (2015) Gestational diabetes: a red flag for future Type 2 diabetes in pregnancy? A retrospective analysis. Diabet Med. doi:10.1111/dme.12723

14. Negrato CA, Gomes MB (2013) Historical facts of screening and diagnosing diabetes in pregnancy. Diabetol Metab Syndr 5:22

15. Thomas CC, Philipson LH (2015) Update on diabetes classification. Med Clin North Am 99:1–16

16. American Diabetes Association (2014) Standards of medical care in diabetes – 2014. Diabetes Care 37(Suppl 1):S14–S80

17. American Diabetes Association (2012) Diagnosis and classification of diabetes mellitus. Diabetes Care 35(Suppl 1):S64–S71

18. Diamond Project Group (2006) Incidence and trends of childhood Type 1 diabetes worldwide 1990–1999. Diabet Med 23:857–866

19. Relimpio F (2003) "The relative contributions of insulin resistance and beta-cell dysfunction to the pathophysiology of Type 2 diabetes", by Kahn SE. Diabetologia 46:1707

20. Feig DS, Zinman B, Wang X, Hux JE (2008) Risk of development of diabetes mellitus after diagnosis of gestational diabetes. CMAJ 179:229–234

21. Bellamy L, Casas JP, Hingorani AD, Williams D (2009) Type 2 diabetes mellitus after gestational diabetes: a systematic review and meta-analysis. Lancet 373:1773–1779

22. Paneni F (2014) 2013 ESC/EASD guidelines on the management of diabetes and cardiovascular disease: established knowledge and evidence gaps. Diab Vasc Dis Res 11:5–10

23. Juarez DT, Demaris KM, Goo R, Mnatzaganian CL, Wong Smith H (2014) Significance of HbA1c and its measurement in the diagnosis of diabetes mellitus: US experience. Diabetes Metab Syndr Obes 7:487–494

24. Xu N, Wu H, Li D, Wang J (2014) Diagnostic accuracy of glycated hemoglobin compared with oral glucose tolerance test for diagnosing diabetes mellitus in Chinese adults: a meta-analysis. Diabetes Res Clin Pract 106:11–18

25. Bartoli E, Fra GP, Carnevale Schianca GP (2011) The oral glucose tolerance test (OGTT) revisited. Eur J Intern Med 22:8–12
26. Ryden L, Grant PJ, Anker SD, Berne C, Cosentino F, Danchin N et al (2013) ESC guidelines on diabetes, pre-diabetes, and cardiovascular diseases developed in collaboration with the EASD: the Task Force on diabetes, pre-diabetes, and cardiovascular diseases of the European Society of Cardiology (ESC) and developed in collaboration with the European Association for the Study of Diabetes (EASD). Eur Heart J 34:3035–3087

Chapter 2
Diabetes and Cardiovascular Disease

2.1 Blood Glucose Levels and Vascular Events

There is a strong biological relation between diabetes mellitus (DM) and cardiovascular disease (CVD) [1]. Several studies make clear that patients with DM are several-fold more likely to develop myocardial infarction and stroke than matched subjects without DM [2, 3]. Metabolic alterations occurring in DM subjects, namely insulin resistance, reduced insulin secretion, or their combination are responsible for endothelial dysfunction, increased platelet reactivity, and inflammation – all factors triggering and accelerating atherosclerotic vascular disease and coronary thrombosis [4, 5]. The detrimental effect of DM on the cardiovascular system is outlined by the fact that 75 % of deaths in DM patients are due to CVD [6]. In a seminal Finnish study, the presence of DM increased the 7-year risk of myocardial infarction and death in older subjects [2]. DM patients also have a three- to sixfold increase in the rate of ischemic cerebrovascular complications [7, 8]. Indeed, T2D was the strongest predictor of ischemic stroke among 16,000 patients enrolled in a prospective Finnish study [9]. More recently, the INTERSTROKE study has demonstrated that DM increases the risk of stroke by 35 %, representing 5 % of the attributable risk for this complication [10]. The analysis of 102

F. Paneni, F. Cosentino, *Diabetes and Cardiovascular Disease:*
A Guide to Clinical Management, DOI 10.1007/978-3-319-17762-5_2,
© Springer International Publishing Switzerland 2015

prospective studies on a total of 698,782 patients has shown that DM patients display a 2.3-fold increase of developing ischemic and hemorrhagic stroke [11]. The concept of DM as a heart disease risk-equivalent emerged from this study and culminated in its coronation as a high-risk cardiovascular state requiring secondary prevention level care [12, 13]. This notion has been further strengthened in the recent 2013 ESC/EASD guidelines on the management of diabetes and CVD [14]. Emerging evidence suggests that the risk of macrovascular complications increases with the severity of abnormality of blood glucose indicating that the relation between metabolic disturbances and vascular damage is approximately linear [15]. Data from the prospective Whitehall study revealed that the risk for CVD was almost doubled in subjects with impaired compared with normal glucose tolerance [16]. The collaborative DECODE study, which analyzed several European cohort studies with baseline OGTT data, showed that mortality was significantly increased in people with DM and IGT, identified by 2hPG, but not in people with IFG [17, 18]. A high 2hPG predicted all-cause and CVD mortality after adjustment for other major CV risk factors, while a high FPG alone was not predictive once 2hPG was taken into account. The follow-up of the *Euro Heart Survey* showed that 1-year survival was significantly higher in prediabetic individuals as compared with DM individuals [19]. However, survival curves tend to overlap in the long-term follow-up, thus strengthening the concept that all stages of glucose abnormalities are associated with increased CV risk [18, 20].

2.2   High Cardiovascular Risk Despite Multifactorial Intervention

Despite clear advances in the prevention and treatment of CVD, the impact of DM on CV outcome remains significantly high and continues to escalate [21]. Even though the cardiovascular

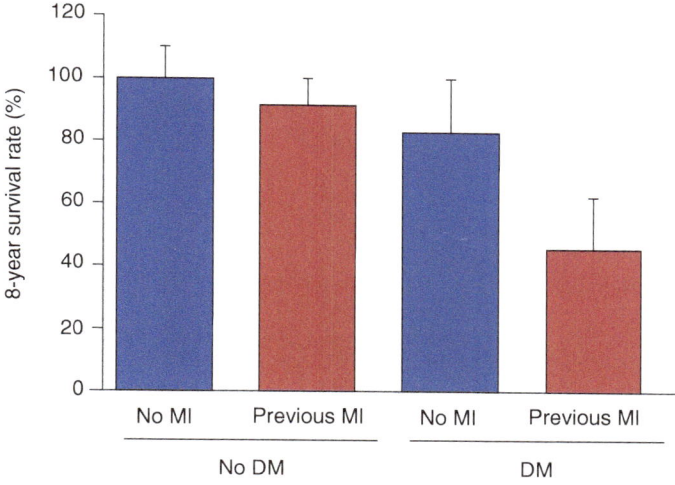

Fig. 2.1 8-year survival rates in patients with myocardial infarction, in the presence or the absence of diabetes mellitus (Modified from Haffner et al. [2])

burden has been reduced over the last decade, this is only partially true in the diabetic patient. In the 10-year follow-up of the NHANES registry (*First National Health and Nutrition Examination Survey*), mortality was significantly lower among non-DM subjects with an acute coronary syndrome (ACS); by contrast such benefit was less evident in diabetic men and women [22]. Moreover, long-term survival (8 years) was dramatically reduced in DM subjects with a previous myocardial infarction as compared with those without DM (Fig. 2.1) [2]. Recent ACS trials such as TIMI-36 and TRITON-TIMI 38 have confirmed that mortality is very high in T2D despite a multifactorial intervention [23, 24]. Consistently, a Danish registry on 3,655 patients with STEMI has confirmed that the rate of myocardial infarction and death is much higher in the

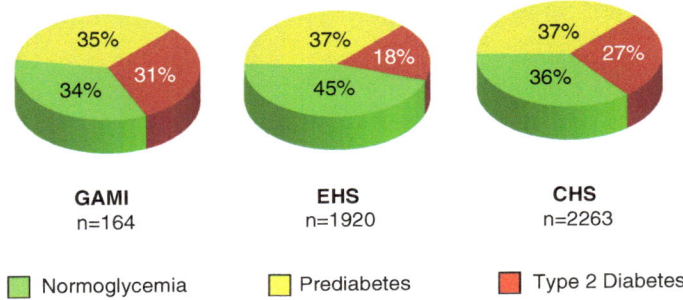

Fig. 2.2 Prevalence of normoglycemia, prediabetes, and diabetes detected by OGTT in patients with coronary artery disease without earlier known diabetes. *EHS* Euro Heart Survey, *CHS* China Heart Survey, *GAMI* Glucose Abnormalities in patients with Myocardial Infarction

presence of DM [25]. Furthermore, the registries EVASTENT and RESTART have shown that the outcome of DM patients is worse even after revascularization, with a substantial increase of stent thrombosis and restenosis [26, 27].

2.3 Impaired Glucose Tolerance in Patients with Coronary Artery Disease

An increasing body of evidence indicates that the prevalence of metabolic disturbances is very high in patients with coronary artery disease without earlier known DM (Fig. 2.2)

[28–30]. In these studies, an OGTT performed at the time of hospital discharge was able to demonstrate that the proportion of patients with IGT was 35 %, whereas 31 % had undetected diabetes earlier. Similar findings were reported in two larger studies, the 25-country *Euro Heart Survey* and the *China Heart Survey* [30, 31]. The *Euro Heart Survey* collected data on European patients ($n = 3{,}444$) with acute and stable coronary artery diseases. Approximately one-third of them ($n = 1{,}524$) had known T2D at study start. An OGTT was performed in 1920 of the patients without known DM, revealing that less than half of them were normoglycemic, 37 % had IGT, and 18 % had unknown DM earlier [30]. The *China Heart Survey*, using the same study design as of the *Euro Heart Survey*, enrolled 3,513 patients with coronary artery disease of whom one-third had established DM earlier. Among the remaining 2,263 patients, OGTTs unveiled DM in 27 % and prediabetes in 37 % [31] (Fig. 2.2). In summary, the evidence for a high prevalence of abnormal glucose metabolism among patients with CVD is strong and universal [32]. This highlights the need for improved strategies for glucometabolic screening and management. Of note, the GAMI study (*Glucose Tolerance in Patients with Acute Myocardial Infarction*) showed that alterations of glucose metabolism detected by OGTT were potent predictors of CV outcome overtime (Fig. 2.3) [29].

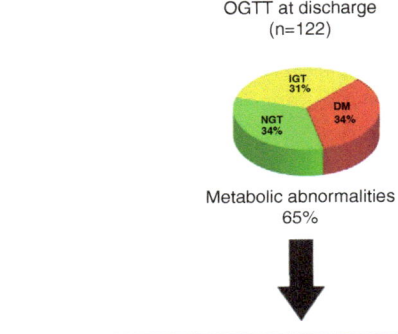

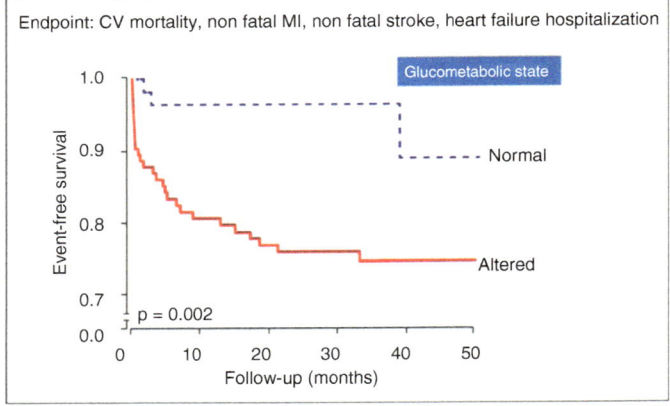

Fig. 2.3 In the GAMI study glucose abnormalities at discharge were an independent predictor of mortality in patients with coronary artery disease. *IGT* impaired glucose tolerance, *NGT* normal glucose tolerance, *DM* diabetes mellitus, *OGTT* oral glucose tolerance test

References

1. Beckman JA, Paneni F, Cosentino F, Creager MA (2013) Diabetes and vascular disease: pathophysiology, clinical consequences, and medical therapy: part II. Eur Heart J 34:2444–2452

2. Haffner SM, Lehto S, Ronnemaa T, Pyorala K, Laakso M (1998) Mortality from coronary heart disease in subjects with type 2 diabetes and in nondiabetic subjects with and without prior myocardial infarction. N Engl J Med 339:229–234

3. Wei M, Gaskill SP, Haffner SM, Stern MP (1998) Effects of diabetes and level of glycemia on all-cause and cardiovascular mortality. The San Antonio Heart Study. Diabetes Care 21:1167–1172

4. Giacco F, Brownlee M (2010) Oxidative stress and diabetic complications. Circ Res 107:1058–1070

5. Paneni F, Beckman JA, Creager MA, Cosentino F (2013) Diabetes and vascular disease: pathophysiology, clinical consequences, and medical therapy: part I. Eur Heart J 34:2436–2443

6. Malmberg K, Yusuf S, Gerstein HC, Brown J, Zhao F, Hunt D et al (2000) Impact of diabetes on long-term prognosis in patients with unstable angina and non-Q-wave myocardial infarction: results of the OASIS (Organization to Assess Strategies for Ischemic Syndromes) Registry. Circulation 102:1014–1019

7. Meschia JF, Bushnell C, Boden-Albala B, Braun LT, Bravata DM, Chaturvedi S et al (2014) Guidelines for the primary prevention of stroke: a statement for healthcare professionals from the American Heart Association/American Stroke Association. Stroke 45:3754–3832

8. Banerjee C, Moon YP, Paik MC, Rundek T, Mora-McLaughlin C, Vieira JR et al (2012) Duration of diabetes and risk of ischemic stroke: the Northern Manhattan Study. Stroke 43:1212–1217

9. Tuomilehto J, Rastenyte D, Jousilahti P, Sarti C, Vartiainen E (1996) Diabetes mellitus as a risk factor for death from stroke. Prospective study of the middle-aged Finnish population. Stroke 27:210–215

10. O'Donnell MJ, Xavier D, Liu L, Zhang H, Chin SL, Rao-Melacini P et al (2010) Risk factors for ischaemic and intracerebral haemorrhagic stroke in 22 countries (the INTERSTROKE study): a case-control study. Lancet 376:112–123

11. Sarwar N, Gao P, Seshasai SR, Gobin R, Kaptoge S, Di Angelantonio E et al (2010) Diabetes mellitus, fasting blood glucose concentration, and risk of vascular disease: a collaborative meta-analysis of 102 prospective studies. Lancet 375:2215–2222

12. Mellbin LG, Anselmino M, Ryden L (2010) Diabetes, prediabetes and cardiovascular risk. Eur J Cardiovasc Prev Rehabil 17(Suppl 1): S9–S14

13. Paneni F (2014) 2013 ESC/EASD guidelines on the management of diabetes and cardiovascular disease: established knowledge and evidence gaps. Diab Vasc Dis Res 11:5–10

14. Ryden L, Grant PJ, Anker SD, Berne C, Cosentino F, Danchin N et al (2013) ESC guidelines on diabetes, pre-diabetes, and cardiovascular diseases developed in collaboration with the EASD: the Task Force on diabetes, pre-diabetes, and cardiovascular diseases of the European Society of Cardiology (ESC) and developed in collaboration with the European Association for the Study of Diabetes (EASD). Eur Heart J 34: 3035–3087

15. Paneni F, Costantino S, Cosentino F (2014) Insulin resistance, diabetes, and cardiovascular risk. Curr Atheroscler Rep 16:419

16. Fuller JH, Shipley MJ, Rose G, Jarrett RJ, Keen H (1980) Coronary-heart-disease risk and impaired glucose tolerance. The Whitehall study. Lancet 1:1373–1376

17. Balkau B (1999) New diagnostic criteria for diabetes and mortality in older adults. DECODE Study Group European Diabetes Epidemiology Group. Lancet 353:68–69

18. The DECODE Study Group. European Diabetes Epidemiology Group. Diabetes Epidemiology: Collaborative analysis Of Diagnostic Criteria in Europe (1999) Glucose tolerance and mortality: comparison of WHO and American Diabetes Association diagnostic criteria. Lancet 354:617–621

19. Lenzen M, Ryden L, Ohrvik J, Bartnik M, Malmberg K, Scholte Op Reimer W et al (2006) Diabetes known or newly detected, but not impaired glucose regulation, has a negative influence on 1-year outcome in patients with coronary artery disease: a report from the Euro Heart Survey on diabetes and the heart. Eur Heart J 27:2969–2974

20. Tominaga M, Eguchi H, Manaka H, Igarashi K, Kato T, Sekikawa A (1999) Impaired glucose tolerance is a risk factor for cardiovascular disease, but not impaired fasting glucose. The Funagata Diabetes Study. Diabetes Care 22:920–924

21. Fioretto P, Dodson PM, Ziegler D, Rosenson RS (2010) Residual microvascular risk in diabetes: unmet needs and future directions. Nat Rev Endocrinol 6:19–25

22. Gu K, Cowie CC, Harris MI (1999) Diabetes and decline in heart disease mortality in US adults. JAMA 281:1291–1297

23. Morrow DA, Scirica BM, Karwatowska-Prokopczuk E, Murphy SA, Budaj A, Varshavsky S et al (2007) Effects of ranolazine on recurrent

cardiovascular events in patients with non-ST-elevation acute coronary syndromes: the MERLIN-TIMI 36 randomized trial. JAMA 297: 1775–1783

24. Wiviott SD, Braunwald E, Angiolillo DJ, Meisel S, Dalby AJ, Verheugt FW et al (2008) Greater clinical benefit of more intensive oral anti-platelet therapy with prasugrel in patients with diabetes mellitus in the trial to assess improvement in therapeutic outcomes by optimizing platelet inhibition with prasugrel-thrombolysis in myocardial infarction 38. Circulation 118:1626–1636

25. Jensen LO, Maeng M, Thayssen P, Tilsted HH, Terkelsen CJ, Kaltoft A et al (2012) Influence of diabetes mellitus on clinical outcomes following primary percutaneous coronary intervention in patients with ST-segment elevation myocardial infarction. Am J Cardiol 109:629–635

26. Machecourt J, Danchin N, Lablanche JM, Fauvel JM, Bonnet JL, Marliere S et al (2007) Risk factors for stent thrombosis after implanta-tion of sirolimus-eluting stents in diabetic and nondiabetic patients: the EVASTENT Matched-Cohort Registry. J Am Coll Cardiol 50: 501–508

27. Kimura T, Morimoto T, Kozuma K, Honda Y, Kume T, Aizawa T et al (2010) Comparisons of baseline demographics, clinical presentation, and long-term outcome among patients with early, late, and very late stent thrombosis of sirolimus-eluting stents: Observations from the Registry of Stent Thrombosis for Review and Reevaluation (RESTART). Circulation 122:52–61

28. Bartnik M, Malmberg K, Hamsten A, Efendic S, Norhammar A, Silveira A et al (2004) Abnormal glucose tolerance – a common risk factor in patients with acute myocardial infarction in comparison with population-based controls. J Intern Med 256:288–297

29. Wallander M, Malmberg K, Norhammar A, Ryden L, Tenerz A (2008) Oral glucose tolerance test: a reliable tool for early detection of glucose abnormalities in patients with acute myocardial infarction in clinical practice: a report on repeated oral glucose tolerance tests from the GAMI study. Diabetes Care 31:36–38

30. Bartnik M, Ryden L, Ferrari R, Malmberg K, Pyorala K, Simoons M et al (2004) The prevalence of abnormal glucose regulation in patients with coronary artery disease across Europe. The Euro Heart Survey on diabetes and the heart. Eur Heart J 25:1880–1890

31. Hu DY, Pan CY, Yu JM (2006) The relationship between coronary artery disease and abnormal glucose regulation in China: the China Heart Survey. Eur Heart J 27:2573–2579

32. Ryden L, Mellbin L (2012) Glucose perturbations and cardiovascular risk: challenges and opportunities. Diab Vasc Dis Res 9:170–176

Chapter 3
Mechanisms of Diabetic Atherosclerosis

3.1 Hyperglycemia, Oxidative Stress, and Endothelial Dysfunction

In patients with diabetes (DM), elevated blood glucose levels exert detrimental effects on endothelial homeostasis, thus precipitating vascular disease phenotypes responsible for adverse cardiovascular events and mortality [1–3]. Chronic hyperglycemia is an independent predictor of macro- and microvascular diabetic complications [2]. In diabetic individuals this condition often clusters with concomitant cardiovascular risk factors such as arterial hypertension, dyslipidemia, and genetic susceptibility, thus amplifying vascular damage [4, 5]. Noteworthy, the detrimental effects of glucose already manifest with glycemic levels below the threshold for the diagnosis of DM. This may be explained by the concept of "glycemic continuum" across the spectrum of prediabetes, diabetes, and cardiovascular risk [6]. Early dysglycemia, a condition commonly observed in subjects with impaired glucose tolerance, plays indeed a key role in triggering pathological processes responsible for atherosclerotic vascular complications [7, 8]. High glucose levels affect vascular homeostasis mostly by altering the balance between nitric oxide (NO) bioavailability and accumulation of reactive oxygen

F. Paneni, F. Cosentino, *Diabetes and Cardiovascular Disease:*
A Guide to Clinical Management, DOI 10.1007/978-3-319-17762-5_3,
© Springer International Publishing Switzerland 2015

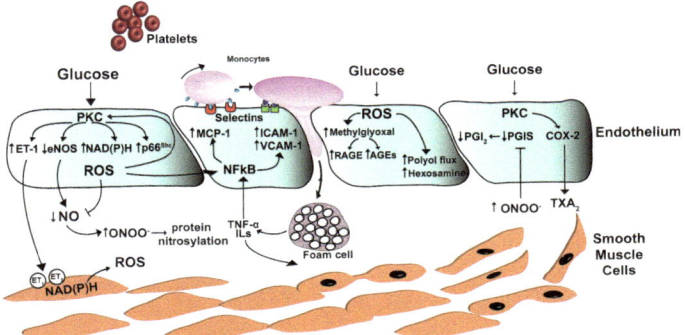

Fig. 3.1 Mechanisms of hyperglycemia-induced vascular damage. *PKC* protein kinase C, *eNOS* endothelial nitric oxide synthase, *ET-1* endothelin 1, *ROS* reactive oxygen species, *NO* nitric oxide, *MCP-1* monocyte chemoattractant protein-1, *VCAM-1* vascular cell adhesion molecule-1, *ICAM-1* intracellular cell adhesion molecule-1, *AGEs* advanced glycation end products

species (ROS) [9, 10]. Accumulation of ROS rapidly inactivates NO to form peroxynitrite (ONOO⁻), a powerful oxidant which easily penetrates across phospholipid membranes thereby suppressing the activity of scavenger enzymes as well as endothelial NO synthase (eNOS, Fig. 3.1). In the diabetic vasculature, oxidative stress is capable to activate an array of cellular pathways including polyol and hexosamine flux, advanced glycation end products (AGEs), protein kinase C (PKC), and NF-kB-mediated vascular inflammation [3, 11]. A recent study showed that PKC is highly activated in endothelial cells isolated from DM subjects and correlates with oxidative stress, impaired insulin signaling, and most importantly endothelial dysfunction as assessed by flow-mediated vasodilation [12]. Once activated, PKC is responsible for different structural and functional changes in the vasculature including alterations of cellular permeability, inflammation, angiogenesis, cell growth, extracellular matrix expansion, and apoptosis [13]. In the diabetic endothelium, PKC leads to increased ROS generation via activation of the adaptor p66[Shc] and NADPH oxidase signaling [14] (Fig. 3.1). The p66[Shc] adaptor protein functions as a redox enzyme implicated in mitochondrial ROS generation and translation of oxidative signals into apoptosis [15]. Notably, p66[Shc] gene expression is increased in peripheral blood mononuclear cells obtained from patients with T2D and correlates with plasma 8-isoprostane levels, an in vivo marker of oxidative stress [16]. Moreover, PKC orchestrates many glucose-sensitive pathways responsible for vasoconstriction and thrombosis such as endothelin-1 and cyclooxigenase-2 (COX-2). In the vessel wall, PKC-dependent ROS production also participates in the atherosclerotic process by triggering vascular inflammation [17]. Indeed, ROS lead to upregulation and nuclear translocation of NF-kB subunit p65 and, hence, transcription of pro-inflammatory genes encoding for monocyte chemoattractant protein-1 (MCP-1), selectins, vascular cell adhesion molecule-1 (VCAM-1), and intracellular cell adhesion molecule-1 (ICAM-1). This latter event facilitates adhesion of monocytes to the vascular endothelium and rolling and diapedesis in the subendothelium with subsequent formation of foam cells [9]. Secretion of IL-1 and TNF-α from active macrophages maintains upregulation of adhesion molecules by enhancing NF-kB signaling in the endothelium and also promotes smooth muscle cell growth and proliferation. Consistently, inhibition of PKC β2 isoform blunts VCAM-1 upregulation in human endothelial cells upon glucose exposure [17]. Mitochondrial ROS also increase intracellular levels of the glucose metabolite methylglyoxal and AGEs synthesis [18, 19]. Generation of AGEs leads to cellular dysfunction by eliciting activation of the AGEs receptor (RAGE). AGE-RAGE signaling in turn activates ROS-sensitive biochemical pathways such as the hexosamine flux [3].

3.2   Insulin Resistance

Insulin resistance (IR) is a major feature of T2D and develops in multiple organs, including skeletal muscle, liver, adipose tissue, and heart. A pooled analysis of 65 trials showed that IR is a strong predictor of coronary heart disease, stroke, or combined CVD (HR 1.64, 1.35–2.00) [20]. Obesity plays a pivotal role in this phenomenon providing an important link between T2D and fat accumulation. In subjects with obesity or T2D, the increase in free fatty acids (FFAs) activate Toll-like receptor 4 (TLR-4) leading to NF-kB nuclear translocation and subsequent up-regulation of inflammatory genes IL-6 and TNF-α. On the other hand, two important kinases, c-Jun amino-terminal kinase (JNK) and PKC, phosphorylate the insulin receptor substrate-1 (IRS-1), thus blunting its downstream targets PI3-kinase and Akt. This results in down-regulation of glucose transporter GLUT-4 and, hence, IR (Fig. 3.2). Although IR has been attributed to adipocyte-derived inflammation, recent evidence is overturning the "adipocentric paradigm" [21]. Indeed, inflammation and macrophage activation seem to primarily occur in nonadipose tissue in obesity. This concept is supported by the notion that suppression of inflammation in the vasculature prevents IR in other organs and prolongs lifespan [22]. Transgenic mice with endothelium-specific overexpression of the inhibitory NF-kB subunit IkBα were protected against the development of IR. In these mice, obesity-induced macrophage infiltration of adipose tissue and plasma oxidative stress markers were reduced whereas blood flow, muscle mitochondrial content, and locomotor activity were increased, confirming the pivotal role of the transcription factor NF-kB in oxidative stress, vascular dysfunction, and inflammation [22]. Another study confirmed these findings, showing that genetic disruption of the insulin receptor substrate 2 (IRS-2) in endothelial cells reduces glucose uptake by the skeletal muscle [23]. These novel findings strengthen the central role of the endothelium in obesity-induced IR, suggesting that blockade of vascular inflammation and oxidative stress may be a promising approach to prevent metabolic disorders.

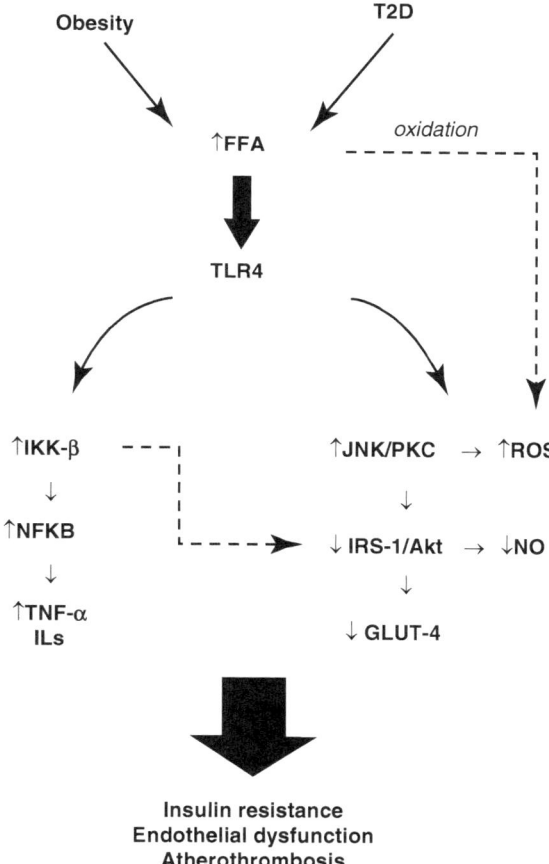

Fig. 3.2 Pathways involved in insulin resistance. *FFA* free fatty acids, *TLR* toll-like receptor, *JNK* c-Jun amino-terminal kinase, *IRS-1* Insulin receptor substrate-1, *NO* nitric oxide, *eNOS* endothelial nitric oxide synthase, *IL-6* interleukin-6, *TNF-α* tumor necrosis factor

Consistently, pharmacological improvement of insulin sensitivity in patients with T2D and metabolic syndrome is associated with restoration of flow-mediated vasodilation [24].

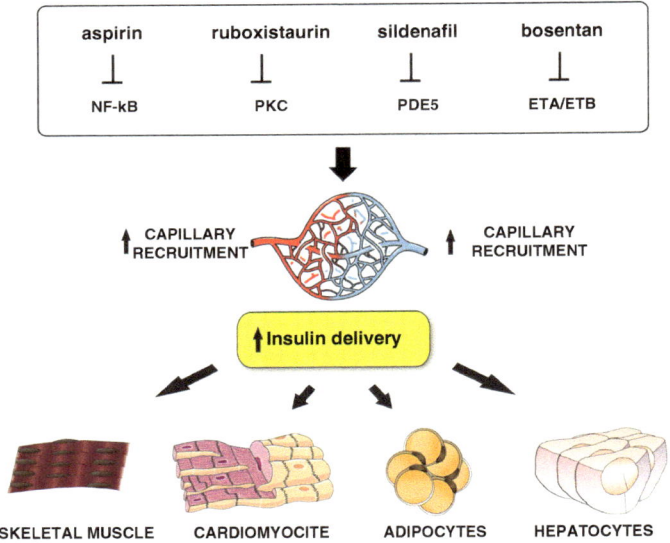

Fig. 3.3 Pharmacological approaches to improve endothelial insulin signaling and systemic glucose tolerance. *NF-kB* nuclear factor kappa-B, *PKC* protein kinase C, *PDE5* phosphodiesterase 5, *ETA/ETB* endothelin receptor A and B

3.3   Molecular Targets to Improve Insulin Sensitivity in Type 2 Diabetes

There are several examples suggesting that mechanism-based therapeutic approaches might be tested to prevent or delay systemic features of IR, favoring adiposity and related comorbidities (Fig. 3.3). High doses of salicylates have been shown to ameliorate IR and improve glucose tolerance by suppressing NF-kB activity in patients with T2D [25]. Moreover, pharmacological inhibition of PKCβ by LY379196 in endothelial cells from T2D patients reduced basal eNOS phosphorylation and improved insulin-mediated eNOS activation [12]. Consistently, the FDA-approved PKC inhibitor ruboxistaurin ameliorates functional endothelial IR and smooth muscle cell hypersensitivity to insulin in experimental obesity and diabetes [26]. The phosphodiesterase 5 (PDE5) inhibitor sildenafil has also shown to improve NOS activity in human endothelial cells exposed to FFAs, suggesting its potential use to improve glucose homeostasis in obese and diabetic subjects [27]. Among different pathways involved, abnormal production and activity of the vasoconstrictor/proatherogenic peptide endothelin-1 (ET-1) is an emerging hallmark of obesity-associated oxidative stress, endothelial dysfunction, inflammation, and altered glucose homeostasis [28]. Insulin resistant states such as T2D, obesity, and arterial hypertension are associated with elevated plasma levels of ET-1 [29]. The vascular responses to ET-1 are mediated via two receptor subtypes: ET_A and ET_B receptors [30]. Both types of receptors are located on vascular smooth muscle cells and mediate vasoconstriction. The ET_B receptor is also located on endothelial cells and mediates vasodilatation by stimulating release of NO and prostacyclin. ET-1 interferes with glucose metabolism as indicated by a drop in splanchnic glucose production and peripheral glucose utilization during ET-1 infusion in healthy subjects [31]. The notion that ET-1 modulates insulin sensitivity is supported by the demonstration that ET-1 induces IR in healthy volunteers [32]. Intravenous infusion of a dual ET_A/ET_B receptor blockade acutely enhances insulin sensitivity in patients with IR and coronary artery disease [33]. Furthermore, preclinical work demonstrated that dual ET_A/ET_B receptor blockade enhanced endothelium-dependent vasodilatation in individuals with IR, suggesting that such an approach may contribute to restore capillary recruitment and insulin delivery to peripheral organs (Fig. 3.3) [34].

3.4   Thrombosis and Coagulation

Coagulation and platelet activation are highly affected in patients with T2D and account for increased risk of coronary events [35]. IR increases PAI-1 and fibrinogen while reducing tPA levels. Hyperinsulinemia and low-grade inflammation induce tissue factor (TF) expression in monocytes of patients with T2D, leading to increased TF procoagulant activity and thrombin generation [36]. Emerging evidence has shown that microparticles (MPs), vesicles released in the circulation from various cell types following activation or apoptosis, are increased in DM patients and predict cardiovascular outcome [37]. MPs carrying TF promote thrombus formation at sites of injury representing a novel and additional mechanism of coronary thrombosis in diabetes [38]. Among the factors contributing to the diabetic prothrombotic state, platelet hyperreactivity is of major relevance [39]. Hyperglycemia alters platelet Ca^{2+} homeostasis leading to cytoskeleton abnormalities and increased secretion of proaggregant factors. Moreover, upregulation of glycoproteins Ib and IIb/IIIa in DM patients triggers thrombus via interacting with von Willebrand factor (vWF) and fibrin molecules (Fig. 3.4) [40].

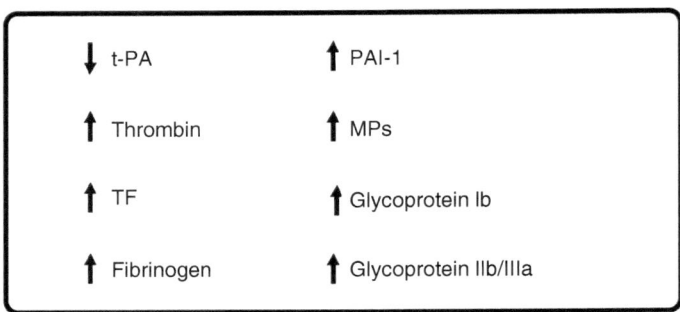

Fig. 3.4 Main alterations of coagulation and platelet functionality in diabetes. *TF* tissue factor, *t-PA* tissue plasminogen activator, *PAI-1* plasminogen activator inhibitor −1, *MPs* microparticles, *vWF* von Willebrand Factor

References

1. Wei M, Gaskill SP, Haffner SM, Stern MP (1998) Effects of diabetes and level of glycemia on all-cause and cardiovascular mortality. The San Antonio Heart Study. Diabetes Care 21:1167–1172
2. Coutinho M, Gerstein HC, Wang Y, Yusuf S (1999) The relationship between glucose and incident cardiovascular events. A metaregression analysis of published data from 20 studies of 95,783 individuals followed for 12.4 years. Diabetes Care 22:233–240
3. Giacco F, Brownlee M (2010) Oxidative stress and diabetic complications. Circ Res 107:1058–1070
4. Paneni F, Costantino S, Cosentino F (2014) Insulin resistance, diabetes, and cardiovascular risk. Curr Atheroscler Rep 16:419
5. DeFronzo RA, Ferrannini E (1991) Insulin resistance. A multifaceted syndrome responsible for NIDDM, obesity, hypertension, dyslipidemia, and atherosclerotic cardiovascular disease. Diabetes Care 14:173–194
6. Mellbin LG, Anselmino M, Ryden L (2010) Diabetes, prediabetes and cardiovascular risk. Eur J Cardiovasc Prev Rehabil 17(Suppl 1):S9–S14
7. Gerstein HC, Pogue J, Mann JFE, Lonn E, Dagenais GR, McQueen M et al (2005) The relationship between dysglycaemia and cardiovascular and renal risk in diabetic and non-diabetic participants in the HOPE study: a prospective epidemiological analysis. Diabetologia 48:1749–1755
8. Sarwar N, Aspelund T, Eiriksdottir G, Gobin R, Seshasai SR, Forouhi NG et al (2010) Markers of dysglycaemia and risk of coronary heart disease in people without diabetes: Reykjavik prospective study and systematic review. PLoS Med 7:e1000278
9. Hink U, Li H, Mollnau H, Oelze M, Matheis E, Hartmann M et al (2001) Mechanisms underlying endothelial dysfunction in diabetes mellitus. Circ Res 88:E14–E22
10. Flammer AJ, Anderson T, Celermajer DS, Creager MA, Deanfield J, Ganz P et al (2012) The assessment of endothelial function: from research into clinical practice. Circulation 126:753–767
11. Nishikawa T, Edelstein D, Du XL, Yamagishi S, Matsumura T, Kaneda Y et al (2000) Normalizing mitochondrial superoxide production blocks three pathways of hyperglycaemic damage. Nature 404:787–790
12. Tabit CE, Shenouda SM, Holbrook M, Fetterman JL, Kiani S, Frame AA et al (2013) Protein kinase C-beta contributes to impaired endothelial insulin signaling in humans with diabetes mellitus. Circulation 127:86–95
13. Geraldes P, King GL (2010) Activation of protein kinase C isoforms and its impact on diabetic complications. Circ Res 106:1319–1331

14. Paneni F, Beckman JA, Creager MA, Cosentino F (2013) Diabetes and vascular disease: pathophysiology, clinical consequences, and medical therapy: part I. Eur Heart J 34:2436–2443

15. Giorgio M, Migliaccio E, Orsini F, Paolucci D, Moroni M, Contursi C et al (2005) Electron transfer between cytochrome c and p66Shc generates reactive oxygen species that trigger mitochondrial apoptosis. Cell 122:221–233

16. Pagnin E, Fadini G, de Toni R, Tiengo A, Calo L, Avogaro A (2005) Diabetes induces p66shc gene expression in human peripheral blood mononuclear cells: relationship to oxidative stress. J Clin Endocrinol Metab 90:1130–1136

17. Kouroedov A, Eto M, Joch H, Volpe M, Luscher TF, Cosentino F (2004) Selective inhibition of protein kinase Cbeta2 prevents acute effects of high glucose on vascular cell adhesion molecule-1 expression in human endothelial cells. Circulation 110:91–96

18. Yan SF, Ramasamy R, Schmidt AM (2010) The RAGE axis: a fundamental mechanism signaling danger to the vulnerable vasculature. Circ Res 106:842–853

19. Jandeleit-Dahm K, Cooper ME (2008) The role of AGEs in cardiovascular disease. Curr Pharm Des 14:979–986

20. Gast KB, Tjeerdema N, Stijnen T, Smit JW, Dekkers OM (2012) Insulin resistance and risk of incident cardiovascular events in adults without diabetes: meta-analysis. PLoS One 7, e52036

21. Kim JK (2012) Endothelial nuclear factor kappaB in obesity and aging: is endothelial nuclear factor kappaB a master regulator of inflammation and insulin resistance? Circulation 125:1081–1083

22. Hasegawa Y, Saito T, Ogihara T, Ishigaki Y, Yamada T, Imai J et al (2012) Blockade of the nuclear factor-kappaB pathway in the endothelium prevents insulin resistance and prolongs life spans. Circulation 125:1122–1133

23. Rask-Madsen C, Li Q, Freund B, Feather D, Abramov R, Wu IH et al (2010) Loss of insulin signaling in vascular endothelial cells accelerates atherosclerosis in apolipoprotein E null mice. Cell Metab 11:379–389

24. Rask-Madsen C, Kahn CR (2012) Tissue-specific insulin signaling, metabolic syndrome, and cardiovascular disease. Arterioscler Thromb Vasc Biol 32:2052–2059

25. Hundal RS, Petersen KF, Mayerson AB, Randhawa PS, Inzucchi S, Shoelson SE et al (2002) Mechanism by which high-dose aspirin improves glucose metabolism in type 2 diabetes. J Clin Invest 109:1321–1326

26. Lu X, Bean JS, Kassab GS, Rekhter MD (2011) Protein kinase C inhibition ameliorates functional endothelial insulin resistance and vascular

smooth muscle cell hypersensitivity to insulin in diabetic hypertensive rats. Cardiovasc Diabetol 10:48

27. Mammi C, Pastore D, Lombardo MF, Ferrelli F, Caprio M, Consoli C et al (2011) Sildenafil reduces insulin-resistance in human endothelial cells. PLoS One 6, e14542

28. Bohm F, Pernow J (2007) The importance of endothelin-1 for vascular dysfunction in cardiovascular disease. Cardiovasc Res 76:8–18

29. Ferri C, Bellini C, Desideri G, Di Francesco L, Baldoncini R, Santucci A et al (1995) Plasma endothelin-1 levels in obese hypertensive and normotensive men. Diabetes 44:431–436

30. Luscher TF, Barton M (2000) Endothelins and endothelin receptor antagonists: therapeutic considerations for a novel class of cardiovascular drugs. Circulation 102:2434–2440

31. Ahlborg G, Weitzberg E, Lundberg JM (1994) Endothelin-1 infusion reduces splanchnic glucose production in humans. J Appl Physiol 77:121–126

32. Ottosson-Seeberger A, Lundberg JM, Alvestrand A, Ahlborg G (1997) Exogenous endothelin-1 causes peripheral insulin resistance in healthy humans. Acta Physiol Scand 161:211–220

33. Ahlborg G, Shemyakin A, Bohm F, Gonon A, Pernow J (2007) Dual endothelin receptor blockade acutely improves insulin sensitivity in obese patients with insulin resistance and coronary artery disease. Diabetes Care 30:591–596

34. Rafnsson A, Bohm F, Settergren M, Gonon A, Brismar K, Pernow J (2012) The endothelin receptor antagonist bosentan improves peripheral endothelial function in patients with type 2 diabetes mellitus and microalbuminuria: a randomised trial. Diabetologia 55:600–607

35. Grant PJ (2007) Diabetes mellitus as a prothrombotic condition. J Intern Med 262:157–172

36. Boden G, Rao AK (2007) Effects of hyperglycemia and hyperinsulinemia on the tissue factor pathway of blood coagulation. Curr Diab Rep 7:223–227

37. Sinning JM, Losch J, Walenta K, Bohm M, Nickenig G, Werner N (2011) Circulating CD31+/Annexin V+ microparticles correlate with cardiovascular outcomes. Eur Heart J 32:2034–2041

38. Tsimerman G, Roguin A, Bachar A, Melamed E, Brenner B, Aharon A (2011) Involvement of microparticles in diabetic vascular complications. Thromb Haemost 106:310–321

39. Linden MD, Tran H, Woods R, Tonkin A (2012) High platelet reactivity and antiplatelet therapy resistance. Semin Thromb Hemost 38:200–212

40. Ferreiro JL, Angiolillo DJ (2011) Diabetes and antiplatelet therapy in acute coronary syndrome. Circulation 123:798–813

Chapter 4
Environment, Epigenetic Changes, and Cardiovascular Damage

4.1 Epigenetic Changes

Environmental cues are potent drivers of altered phenotypes and disease states. Exposure to different stimuli may indeed favor detrimental changes eliciting pathological processes in different organs, thus precipitating a cluster of comorbidities such as obesity, diabetes (DM), and cardiovascular disease (CVD) [1, 2]. These conditions often occur simultaneously and significantly aggravate human health by affecting quality of life as well as lifespan [3]. Insightful epigenetic analyses are revealing that gene-activating events occurring in obese subjects are transmitted to the offspring [4, 5]. Inheritance of these modifications may anticipate disease phenotypes already in young, normoweight individuals [5]. Therefore, transmission of metabolic signatures over the next generations implicates an exponential increase of obesity-related disorders, with a further rise of morbidity [6]. Recent evidence indicates that epigenetic changes may contribute to explain gene-environment interaction and subsequent dysregulation of critical pathways involved in diabetic vascular disease phenotype [7]. Epigenetics refers to heritable changes in gene expression without altering the DNA sequence [8]. Epigenetic variations may be classified into three

F. Paneni, F. Cosentino, *Diabetes and Cardiovascular Disease:*
A Guide to Clinical Management, DOI 10.1007/978-3-319-17762-5_4,
© Springer International Publishing Switzerland 2015

main categories: (1) DNA methylation, (2) posttranslational histone modifications, and (3) RNA-based mechanisms including microRNAs and long noncoding RNAs.

4.2   DNA Methylation and Histone Modifications

Chromatin is composed by chromosomal DNA packaged around histone proteins known as nucleosomes. A nucleosome has 147 base pairs of DNA wrapped around an octomeric core of proteins, which consists of two H3–H4 histone dimers surrounded by two H2A–H2B dimers [7, 8]. Histones and DNA are tightly linked by multiple interactions which make nucleosomes very stable under physiological conditions. The nucleosome is a complex structure amenable of plastic changes which are governed by an array of protein complexes. These modifications are highly relevant since dynamic changes of chromatin structure strongly affect almost all DNA-related processes including transcription, recombination, DNA repair, and replication [9]. The major mechanisms of epigenetic regulation are represented by DNA methylation of cytosine-paired-with-guanine (CpG) dinucleotide sequences as well as methylation or acetylation of histone proteins. DNA methylation is an important repressor of gene transcription and refers to the covalent attachment of a methyl group to cytosine residues in CpG islands. Posttranslational modification of histone tails (acetylation/methylation) also represent key components in the epigenetic regulation of genes. Several enzymes have been implicated in plastic alterations of chromatin upon physiological and pathological conditions [10]. DNA and histone methyltransferases (DNMTs and HMTs), as well as histone acetyltransferases (HATs), orchestrate a fine balance between activating and inhibitory epigenetic signatures (Fig. 4.1).

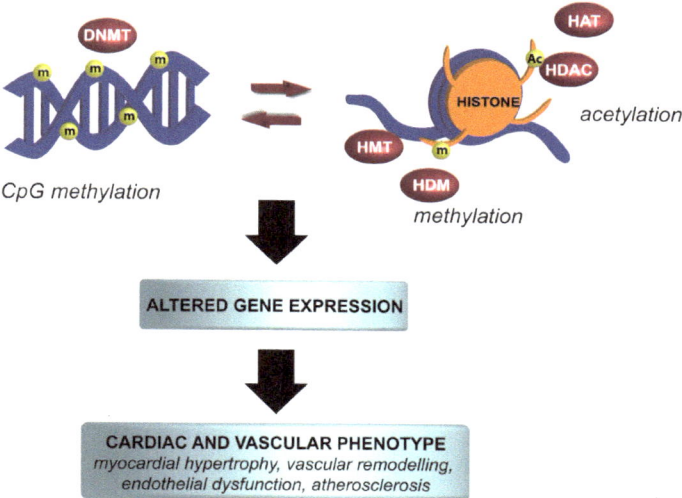

Fig. 4.1 Modification of DNA/histone complexes as triggers of cardiovascular disease. *DNMT* DNA methyltransferase, *HATs* histone acetyltransferase, *HDAC* histone deacetylase, *HM* histone methylase, *HDM* histone demethylase. Ac and m indicate acetylation and methylation of histone tails

4.3   Chromatin Remodeling and Diabetic Atherosclerosis

In 2008, El-Osta et al. found that transient hyperglycemia in aortic endothelial cells was able to induce long-lasting epigenetic changes in the promoter of the nuclear factor κB (NF-κB) subunit p65 [11]. This epigenetic deregulation explains persistent p65 gene transcription and subsequent overexpression of the inflammatory genes monocyte chemoattractant protein-1 (MCP-1) and vascular cell adhesion molecule-1 (VCAM-1) after 6 days of glucose normalization. Interestingly, normalization of mitochondrial superoxide production dislodged the epigenetic markers at p65 promoter, clearly indicating that ROS still remain the upstream key molecules involved in the pathophysiology of diabetic vascular disease despite glucose control. Indeed, hyperglycemia-dependent ROS production was responsible for monomethylation of histone 3 at lysine 4 amino residue (H3K4m) by the mammalian methyltransferase Set7/9. Methylation of H3K4 is a critical posttranslational modification favoring gene transcription in mammals and is associated with persistent vascular inflammation when such methylation occurs on histone 3 binding the proximal promoter region of NF-κB subunit p65 [12, 13]. Interestingly, knockdown of Set7/9 prevented H3K4m and, hence, glucose-induced upregulation of p65 as well as of MCP-1 and VCAM-1 genes (Fig. 4.2) [11]. This study demonstrated that overproduction of ROS leads to activation of key enzymes involved in chromatin remodeling and persistent transcription of inflammatory genes. We have recently showed that expression of Set7 is increased in peripheral blood monocytes isolated from diabetic patients [14]. T2D patients showed Set7-dependent H3K4m on NF-kB p65 promoter and this epigenetic signature was associated with upregulation of NF-kB p65, subsequent transcription of oxidant genes (iNOS and COX-2) and increased plasma levels of ICAM-1 and MCP-1. Consistently, Set7 expression significantly correlated with oxidative marker 8-isoPGF$_2$α and flow-mediated dilation of the brachial artery [14]. These findings in humans show that Set7 may represent a promising target to prevent atherosclerotic vascular disease in the context of cardiometabolic disturbances. Other studies revealed further molecular networks linking chromatin modifying enzymes with NF-kB signaling. Vascular smooth muscle cells (VSMCs) from db/db mice showed decreased expression of the methyltransferase Suv39h1 and increased LSD1 activity on the NF-kB p65 promoter, leading to suppression of dimethylation (H3K9m2) and trimethylation of H3 at lysine 9 (H3K9m3) bound to the promoters of inflammatory

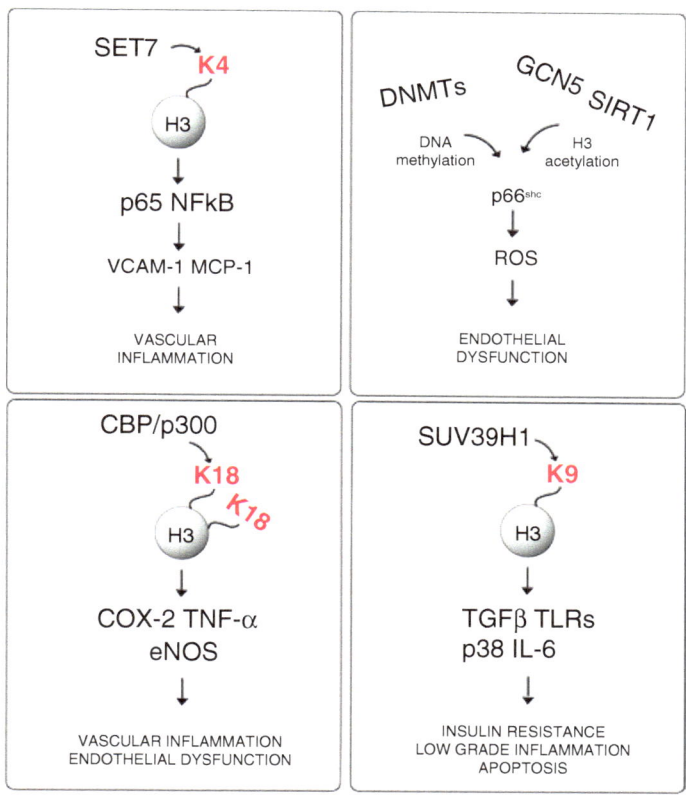

Fig. 4.2 Main epigenetic networks associated with diabetes. *DNMTs* DNA methyltransferase, *H3* histone 3, *ROS* reactive oxygen species, *K* lysine residue, *COX-2* cycloxygenase-2, *TNF-α* tumor necrosis factor- α, *eNOS* endothelial nitric oxide synthase, *TGFβ* transforming growth factor β, *TLRs* Toll-like receptors, *NF-kB* nuclear factor KB, *VCAM-1* vascular cell adhesion molecule-1, *MCP-1* monocyte chemotactic protein-1

genes (IL-6 and MCP-1) [15]. Interestingly, overexpression of Suv39h1 reversed the diabetic phenotype in VSMCs while knockdown of this methyltransferase increased the expression of inflammatory genes. We have recently found that epigenetic regulation of the mitochondrial adaptor p66[Shc], a key enzyme involved in mitochondrial ROS generation, may significantly contribute to endothelial dysfunction in the context of diabetes [16]. Specifically, promoter CpG demethylation and H3 acetylation were responsible for persistent p66[Shc] upregulation, even after restoration of normoglycemia. This latter modification were mediated by deregulation of methyltransferase DNMT and acetyltransferase general control nonderepressible 5 (Gcn5). Indeed, downregulation or pharmacological inhibition of Gcn5 blunted persistent p66[Shc] overexpression (Fig. 4.2) [16]. Recent evidence suggest the important role of histone acetyltransferases (HATs) and histone deacetylases (HDACs) in the regulation of several genes linked to endothelial dysfunction and inflammation in diabetes [17]. Interestingly, the sirtuin family of deacetylases has been found to regulate several factors involved in metabolism, adipogenesis, and insulin secretion [18, 19]. Moreover, a recent study reported that vascular p66[Shc] gene transcription is epigenetically regulated by SIRT1 [20]. Specifically, SIRT1 decreases acetylation of H3 binding p66[Shc] promoter. Overexpression of this sirtuin inhibited high glucose-induced p66[Shc] upregulation whereas its knockdown exerted opposite effects. In line with these findings, SIRT1 activation blunts ROS formation, suppressing NF-kB activation and cleavage of poly (ADP-ribose) polymerase (PARP). HATs and HDACs can also modulate NF-kB transcriptional activity, resulting in changes in downstream inflammatory gene expression levels. Interestingly, high glucose treatment of cultured monocytes increased recruitment of the HATs CPB and p/CAF, leading to increased histone lysine acetylation at the cyclooxygenase-2 (COX-2) and TNF-α inflammatory gene promoters [21]. Monocyte expression of inflammatory cytokines in response to high glucose concentrations requires the interaction between NFκB and HATs, leading to hyperacetylation and transcriptional activation. Methylation of H3K9 is known to repress genes relevant to autoimmune and inflammatory pathways in lymphocytes from patients with type 1 diabetes [22]. Indeed, silencing of the H3K9 methylation-writing enzyme SUV39H1 in human smooth muscle cells increased the expression of inflammatory genes [23]. Taken together, these studies suggest that the removal of epigenetic marks of oxidant and inflammatory genes may represent a promising option to prevent endothelial dysfunction and, hence, vascular complications in people with diabetes.

4.4 Epigenetic Inheritance

Epigenetic inheritance is an attractive theory to explain the rising prevalence of cardiometabolic disturbances which can be transmitted throughout multiple generations [24]. In animals, it has been demonstrated that long-term exposure to a methyl donor rich diet for six generations results in a large number of loci exhibiting epigenetic variability, suggesting that some of the induced changes are heritable [25]. Another study in mice fed high fed diet (HFD) showed that obesity occurs earlier and becomes more severe through generations (F2 > F1 > F0) [26]. Moreover, this phenomenon was accompanied by a gradual increase of histological scoring of hepatic steatosis in male mice with transgenerational HFD feeding. Interestingly, the highest degree of steatosis occurred in HFD-treated F2 mice and was associated with the highest levels of insulin and leptin. As a consequence the latter, mice were characterized by enhanced lipogenesis and endoplasmic reticulum stress, important biochemical fingerprints of insulin resistance. Other studies found that the metabolic effects of maternal HFD exposure on body length and insulin insensitivity persist across at least two generations of

offspring [27]. A recent work showed that epigenetic modifications induced by hyperglycemia are transmitted to the offspring
even after restoration of normoglycemic conditions [28]. Hence,
glucose normalization in adult diabetic zebrafish was not sufficient to prevent inheritance of detrimental epigenetic signatures
in the daughter tissue, suggesting that the so-called metabolic
memory is an inheritable phenomenon. Indeed, CpG island
methylation and genome-wide microarray expression analyses
revealed the persistence of hyperglycemia-induced global DNA
hypomethylation that correlated with aberrant gene expression
for a subset of loci in the offspring [28]. However, further
research is warranted to confirm whether these mechanisms can
be translated to diabetic patients. In humans, longitudinal studies
have demonstrated that DM during pregnancy is followed by
markedly increased rates of offspring obesity, as well as premature incidence of T2D [10]. Moreover, offspring of DM women
display an increased risk of DM, and epigenetic modifications
are certainly involved in this phenomenon [29]. Strong evidence
supporting the impact of early nutritional environment comes
from well-studied cohorts of men and women who were exposed
in utero to the Dutch famine of 1944–1945 [30]. These subjects
showed subtle blood methylation changes of insulin-like growth
factor-2 (IGF-2) and leptin (Lep) genes. Interestingly, they had
an increased risk for cardiometabolic disease, accelerated cognitive aging, and schizophrenia [6]. Furthermore, the observed
neonatal adiposity suggests a possible transgenerational effect of
maternal undernutrition.

4.5   MicroRNAs

MicroRNAs (miRs) are a newly identified class of small noncoding RNAs emerging as key players in the pathogenesis of
diabetes-induced vascular complications [31]. These noncoding

RNAs trigger diabetic vascular disease by regulating gene expression at the posttranscriptional level. Microarray studies have shown an altered profile of miRs expression in subjects with T2D [32, 33]. Indeed, DM patients display a significant deregulation of miRs involved in angiogenesis, vascular repair, and endothelial homeostasis [32]. Over the last few years, different studies have explored the mechanisms whereby deregulation of miRs expression may contribute to vascular disease in subjects with DM. Table 4.1 shows the main miRs found in DM and their mechanism of action. In endothelial cells exposed to high glucose, miR-320 is highly expressed and targets several angiogenic factors and their receptors, including vascular endothelial growth factor (VEGF) and insulin-like growth factor-1 (IGF-1) [34]. Elevated levels of this miR are associated with decreased cell proliferation and migration, while its downregulation restores these properties and increases IGF-1 expression, promoting angiogenesis and vascular repair. Hyperglycemia also increases the expression of miR-221, a regulator of angiogenesis targeting the receptor for stem cells factor c-kit (CD117) responsible for migration and homing of endothelial progenitor cells (EPCs) [35]. A recent study demonstrated that miR-503 is critically involved in hyperglycemia-induced endothelial dysfunction in diabetic mice and is upregulated in ischemic limb muscles of diabetic subjects [36]. The detrimental effects of miR-503 in the setting of DM have been explained by its interaction with CCNE and cdc25A, critical regulators of cell cycle progression affecting endothelial cell migration and proliferation. Interestingly, miR-503 inhibition was able to normalize postischemic neovascularization and blood flow recovery in diabetic mice. Plasma microRNA profiling showed a profound downregulation of miR-126 in a cohort of DM patients [32]. Recent evidence suggest that reduced miR-126 expression levels are partially responsible for impaired vascular repair capacities in DM [37]. Collectively, these studies support the notion that miRs drive complex

Table 4.1   Principal microRNAs and their relative target genes contributing to reduced vascular repair and, hence, diabetes-related vascular dysfunction

MicroRNA	Expression	Molecular target	Biological effect
miR-320	Increased	VEGF/IGF-1	Impaired angiogenesis
miR-221	Increased	c-kit	Reduced proliferation, migration, and homing of EPCs
miR-222	Decreased	P27KIP1/P57KIP2	AGEs synthesis
miR-503	Increased	CCNE/cdc25A	Reduced angiogenesis, endothelial dysfunction
miR-126	Decreased	Spred-1	Reduced EPCs functionality and angiogenesis

VEGF vascular endothelial growth factor, *IGF-1* insulin-like growth factor-1, *AGEs* advanced glycation end products

signaling networks by targeting the expression of genes involved in cell differentiation, migration, and survival (Table 4.1).

References

1. Skinner MK (2014) Environment, epigenetics and reproduction. Mol Cell Endocrinol 398:1–3
2. Steves CJ, Spector TD, Jackson SH (2012) Ageing, genes, environment and epigenetics: what twin studies tell us now, and in the future. Age Ageing 41:581–586
3. Bollati V, Baccarelli A (2010) Environmental epigenetics. Heredity 105:105–112

4. Skinner MK, Guerrero-Bosagna C (2009) Environmental signals and transgenerational epigenetics. Epigenomics 1:111–117
5. Bouret S, Levin BE, Ozanne SE (2015) Gene-environment interactions controlling energy and glucose homeostasis and the developmental origins of obesity. Physiol Rev 95:47–82
6. Napoli C, Crudele V, Soricelli A, Al-Omran M, Vitale N, Infante T et al (2012) Primary prevention of atherosclerosis: a clinical challenge for the reversal of epigenetic mechanisms? Circulation 125:2363–2373
7. Keating ST, El-Osta A (2015) Epigenetics and Metabolism. Circ Res 116:715–736
8. Handy DE, Castro R, Loscalzo J (2011) Epigenetic modifications: basic mechanisms and role in cardiovascular disease. Circulation 123: 2145–2156
9. Henikoff S, Smith MM (2015) Histone variants and epigenetics. Cold Spring Harb Perspect Biol 7:a019364
10. Paneni F, Costantino S, Volpe M, Luscher TF, Cosentino F (2013) Epigenetic signatures and vascular risk in type 2 diabetes: a clinical perspective. Atherosclerosis 230:191–197
11. El-Osta A, Brasacchio D, Yao D, Pocai A, Jones PL, Roeder RG et al (2008) Transient high glucose causes persistent epigenetic changes and altered gene expression during subsequent normoglycemia. J Exp Med 205:2409–2417
12. Keating ST, El-Osta A (2012) Chromatin modifications associated with diabetes. J Cardiovasc Transl Res 5:399–412
13. Li Y, Reddy MA, Miao F, Shanmugam N, Yee JK, Hawkins D et al (2008) Role of the histone H3 lysine 4 methyltransferase, SET7/9, in the regulation of NF-kappaB-dependent inflammatory genes. Relevance to diabetes and inflammation. J Biol Chem 283:26771–26781
14. Paneni F, Costantino S, Battista R, Castello L, Capretti G, Chiandotto S et al (2015) Adverse epigenetic signatures by histone methyltransferase set7 contribute to vascular dysfunction in patients with type 2 diabetes mellitus. Circ Cardiovasc Genet 8:150–158
15. Li SL, Reddy MA, Cai Q, Meng L, Yuan H, Lanting L et al (2006) Enhanced proatherogenic responses in macrophages and vascular smooth muscle cells derived from diabetic db/db mice. Diabetes 55:2611–2619
16. Paneni F, Mocharla P, Akhmedov A, Costantino S, Osto E, Volpe M et al (2012) Gene silencing of the mitochondrial adaptor p66(Shc) suppresses vascular hyperglycemic memory in diabetes. Circ Res 111:278–289
17. Cooper ME, El-Osta A (2010) Epigenetics: mechanisms and implications for diabetic complications. Circ Res 107:1403–1413

18. Paneni F, Volpe M, Luscher TF, Cosentino F (2013) SIRT1, p66Shc, and Set7/9 in vascular hyperglycemic memory: bringing all the strands together. Diabetes 62:1800–1807

19. Corbi G, Conti V, Scapagnini G, Filippelli A, Ferrara N (2012) Role of sirtuins, calorie restriction and physical activity in aging. Front Biosci 4:768–778

20. Zhou S, Chen HZ, Wan YZ, Zhang QJ, Wei YS, Huang S et al (2011) Repression of P66Shc expression by SIRT1 contributes to the prevention of hyperglycemia-induced endothelial dysfunction. Circ Res 109:639–648

21. Miao F, Gonzalo IG, Lanting L, Natarajan R (2004) In vivo chromatin remodeling events leading to inflammatory gene transcription under diabetic conditions. J Biol Chem 279:18091–18097

22. Miao F, Smith DD, Zhang L, Min A, Feng W, Natarajan R (2008) Lymphocytes from patients with type 1 diabetes display a distinct profile of chromatin histone H3 lysine 9 dimethylation: an epigenetic study in diabetes. Diabetes 57:3189–3198

23. Villeneuve LM, Reddy MA, Lanting LL, Wang M, Meng L, Natarajan R (2008) Epigenetic histone H3 lysine 9 methylation in metabolic memory and inflammatory phenotype of vascular smooth muscle cells in diabetes. Proc Natl Acad Sci USA 105:9047–9052

24. Szyf M (2015) Nongenetic inheritance and transgenerational epigenetics. Trends Mol Med 21:134–144

25. Li CC, Cropley JE, Cowley MJ, Preiss T, Martin DI, Suter CM (2011) A sustained dietary change increases epigenetic variation in isogenic mice. PLoS Genet 7:e1001380

26. Li J, Huang J, Li JS, Chen H, Huang K, Zheng L (2012) Accumulation of endoplasmic reticulum stress and lipogenesis in the liver through generational effects of high fat diets. J Hepatol 56:900–907

27. Dunn GA, Bale TL (2009) Maternal high-fat diet promotes body length increases and insulin insensitivity in second-generation mice. Endocrinology 150:4999–5009

28. Olsen AS, Sarras MP Jr, Leontovich A, Intine RV (2012) Heritable transmission of diabetic metabolic memory in zebrafish correlates with DNA hypomethylation and aberrant gene expression. Diabetes 61:485–491

29. Brasset E, Chambeyron S (2013) Epigenetics and transgenerational inheritance. Genome Biol 14:306

30. Roseboom TJ, Painter RC, van Abeelen AF, Veenendaal MV, de Rooij SR (2011) Hungry in the womb: what are the consequences? Lessons from the Dutch famine. Maturitas 70:141–145

31. Shantikumar S, Caporali A, Emanueli C (2012) Role of microRNAs in diabetes and its cardiovascular complications. Cardiovasc Res 93:583–593

32. Zampetaki A, Kiechl S, Drozdov I, Willeit P, Mayr U, Prokopi M et al (2010) Plasma microRNA profiling reveals loss of endothelial miR-126 and other microRNAs in type 2 diabetes. Circ Res 107:810–817

33. Karolina DS, Armugam A, Tavintharan S, Wong MT, Lim SC, Sum CF et al (2011) MicroRNA 144 impairs insulin signaling by inhibiting the expression of insulin receptor substrate 1 in type 2 diabetes mellitus. PLoS One 6:e22839

34. Wang XH, Qian RZ, Zhang W, Chen SF, Jin HM, Hu RM (2009) MicroRNA-320 expression in myocardial microvascular endothelial cells and its relationship with insulin-like growth factor-1 in type 2 diabetic rats. Clin Exp Pharmacol Physiol 36:181–188

35. Li Y, Song YH, Li F, Yang T, Lu YW, Geng YJ (2009) MicroRNA-221 regulates high glucose-induced endothelial dysfunction. Biochem Biophys Res Commun 381:81–83

36. Caporali A, Meloni M, Vollenkle C, Bonci D, Sala-Newby GB, Addis R et al (2011) Deregulation of microRNA-503 contributes to diabetes mellitus-induced impairment of endothelial function and reparative angiogenesis after limb ischemia. Circulation 123:282–291

37. Mocharla P, Briand S, Giannotti G, Dorries C, Jakob P, Paneni F et al (2013) AngiomiR-126 expression and secretion from circulating CD34(+) and CD14(+) PBMCs: role for proangiogenic effects and alterations in type 2 diabetics. Blood 121:226–236

Chapter 5
Diabetic Cardiomyopathy

5.1 Heart Failure in Patients with Diabetes

Patients with diabetes (DM) have a high risk of left ventricular dysfunction (LVD) and heart failure (HF) as compared with non-DM subjects. In the Framingham study, DM men and women had a six- to eightfold increase in the prevalence of HF, with the highest number of cases observed in the latter group. Among patients with HF, 15–25 % have DM, a condition which amplifies morbidity and mortality [1]. The SOLVD study (*Studies of Left Ventricular Dysfunction*) has shown that 15–26 % of patients with LVD had DM at the time of enrolment [2]. The V-Heft and, more recently, the ATLAS study showed that the proportion of DM patients with HF may reach 20 % [3, 4]. Interestingly, risk of HF already increases in non-DM patients with impaired glucose tolerance. This notion is supported by seminal studies showing that insulin resistance, detected by glycemic-hyperinsulinemic clamp, is strongly and independently associated with incidence of HF, with more than 20 persons/year affected in the lowest clamp quartile [5]. In this study, fasting plasma glucose, OGTT 2 h glucose, and waist

F. Paneni, F. Cosentino, *Diabetes and Cardiovascular Disease:*
A Guide to Clinical Management, DOI 10.1007/978-3-319-17762-5_5,
© Springer International Publishing Switzerland 2015

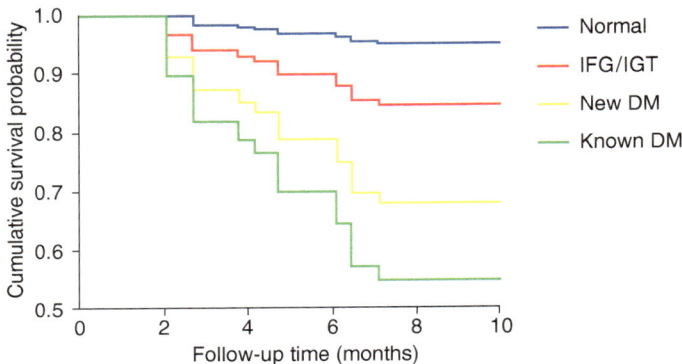

Fig. 5.1 Kaplan-Meier survival curve for all-cause mortality stratified by glucose metabolism. Log-rank: p 0.001. *IFG* impaired fasting glucose, *IGT* impaired glucose tolerance, *DM* diabetes (Modified with permission from Hofsten et al. [6])

circumference were all associated with incident HF, suggesting that metabolic traits significantly increase the susceptibility to develop myocardial dysfunction. Moreover, IFG/IGT, new onset DM and known DM were linked to a progressive increase of death or hospitalization for HF (Fig. 5.1) [6]. Collectively, these data support the concept of the glycemic continuum and indicate that the relation between glucose abnormalities and HF is almost linear.

5.2   Diastolic Dysfunction

Although DM is strongly associated with coronary artery disease (CAD), many cases of LVD occur in subjects with nonobstructive CAD. These data suggest that DM per se is sufficient to impair cardiac performance by affecting ventricular

Peripheral edema

Dyspnea

Low-normal EF (45–50 %)

Diastolic dysfunction (pseudonormal filling pattern)

Increased atrial volume

Eccentric hypertrophy

Increased vena cava diameter

Mild, diffuse coronary artery disease

Fig. 5.2 Main clinical features of patients presenting with diabetic cardio-myopathy. *EF* ejection fraction

structure and function. This notion has been documented by autopsies showing that the diabetic heart is characterized by myocardial fibrosis, left ventricular hypertrophy, eccentric remodeling pattern, and capillary microaneurysms [7]. Myocardial stiffness with reduced compliance precipitates diastolic dysfunction with a progressive increase of LV filling pressures and diastolic heart failure (DHF) [8]. Indeed, many DM patients present at the emergency department with signs of HF which are mostly explained by defects of diastolic function whereas systolic performance is preserved [9]. A typical clinical presentation is characterized by progressive exertional dyspnea and mild lower-extremity edema. Transthoracic echocardiogram usually reveals moderate LV hypertrophy, low-normal ejection fraction (45–50 %), pseudonormal diastolic filling, and a dilated inferior vena cava (Fig. 5.2). These features explain why a large part of HF cases in DM patients is characterized by a severe impairment of diastolic function whereas systolic performance is still preserved [10]. Indeed, patients with DM have a higher risk of diastolic than systolic HF with hazard rations of 1.12 (1.06–1.18, $p < 0.001$) and 1.07 (0.02–1.12, <0.01), respectively [11]. Notably, prospective analyses have shown that the prognosis of DHF is comparable to the one reported for patients with reduced systolic function, with a 50–60 % mortality rate after 5 years [11]. DM patients with DHF often display pronounced alterations of metabolic parameters including poor glycemic control (HbA1c >7.5 %), hypertension, and atherogenic dysplidemia with particular increase of triglycerides [12]. The latter aspects are responsible for another important pathological feature of the diabetic heart, known as cardiac myocyte steatosis [13, 14].

5.3   Lipotoxicity

Accumulation of circulating fatty acids is one of the main biochemical events favoring disturbances of signaling pathways in the diabetic heart [14, 15]. The heart of DM patients is indeed bathed in elevated concentrations of FFAs and glucose. Human studies using positron emission tomography tracers have reproducibly demonstrated increased basal FFAs oxidation coupled with decreased myocardial glucose oxidation in patients with obesity and DM [16]. The heart is a metabolically flexible organ, which has the ability to quickly shift its substrate to maintain normal ATP levels. In the insulin resistant myocardium, the decrease in glucose oxidation is compensated by FFAs oxidation via an array of transcriptional programs mostly driven by nuclear receptor transcription factor-alpha (PPARα) (Fig. 5.3) [17]. This complex regulates many genes favoring metabolic flexibility though fatty acids import, fatty acids oxidation, and triglyceride synthesis. Moreover, PPARα hampers glucose oxidation by upregulating PDK4, which prevents the entry of glucose into the citric acid cycle. Beside these biochemical effects, activation of NF-kB pathway in the diabetic myocardium leads to downregulation of GLUT4 with subsequent reduction of glucose uptake and amplification of FFAs-induced insulin resistance [15, 18]. Oxidation of FFAs, as many compensatory mechanisms, shows high efficiency in the short-term while it becomes maladaptive with time. Indeed, prolonged FFAs oxidation triggers excessive mitochondrial ROS production, less efficient energy generation, and the production of incompletely oxidized acyl-carnitine metabolites and toxic lipid species [19]. Accumulation of intracellular lipids may also directly contribute to cell death. Reaction of palmityol-CoA with serine leads to the generation of ceramide, a sphingolipid which can trigger myocyte apoptosis through inhibition of the mitochondrial respiratory chain (Fig. 5.3).

5.4 Glucotoxicity

Glucotoxicity represents another detrimental mechanism of myocardial damage in DM. Hyperglycemia, a consequence of decreased glucose clearance and augmented hepatic gluconeogenesis, triggers mitochondrial reactive oxygen species (ROS) by activating different signaling cascades including protein kinase C (PKC), NADPH oxidase, hexosamine, and polyol pathways as well as advanced glycation end products (AGEs) (Fig. 5.3). Hyperactive PKC signaling in the heart can influence calcium handling, ROS generation, and inflammation, all of which can affect cardiac performance [20–23]. Indeed, transgenic mice with cardiac overexpression of PKCβ develop cardiomyopathy [24]. Moreover, other evidence suggests that PKCβ inhibition can improve the cardiac phenotype of STZ-injected rats [20]. PKCβ can amplify oxidative damage by

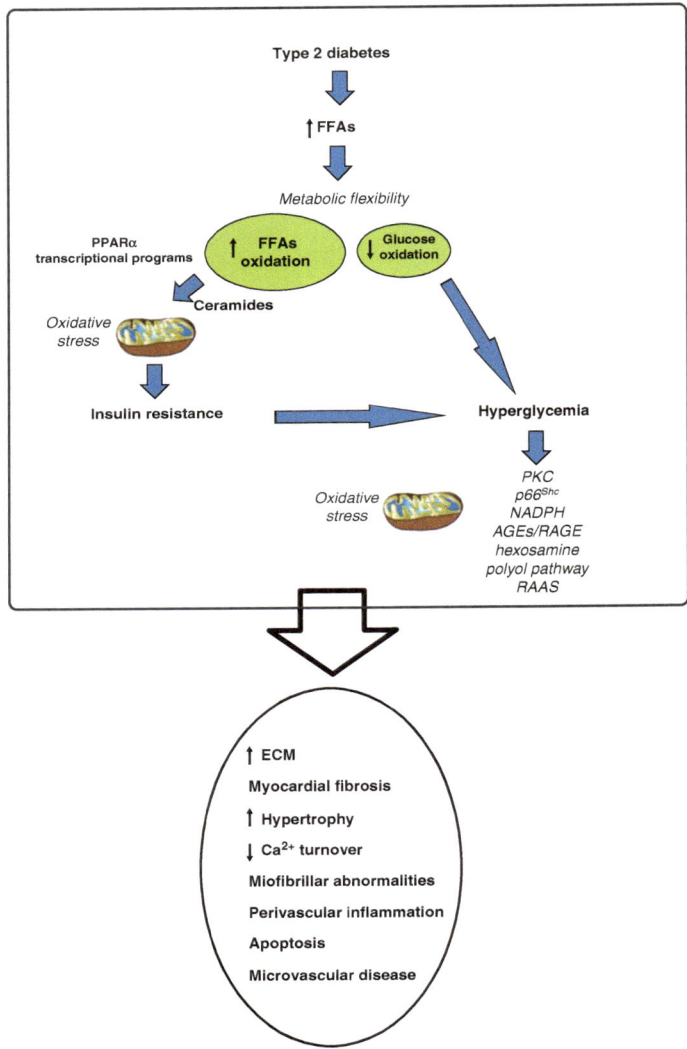

Fig. 5.3 Molecular mechanisms of diabetic cardiomyopathy. *FFAs* free fatty acids, *PPARα* peroxisome proliferator-activated receptor alpha, *PKC* protein kinase C, *AGE* advanced glycation end-productions, *RAGE* AGE receptor, *ECM* extracellular matrix

phosphorylating NADPH subunit p47phox as well as the mitochondrial adaptor p66[Shc], a key enzyme involved in ROS generation, mitochondrial disruption, and cellular apoptosis [25]. ROS-induced apoptosis activates poly (ADPribose) polymerase-1 (PARP). This enzyme mediates the direct ribosylation and inhibition of glyceraldehyde phosphate dehydrogenase (GAPDH), diverting glucose from the glycolytic pathway toward alternative biochemical cascades that participate to hyperglycemia-induced cellular injury [26]. High glucose levels also activate tissue renin angiotensin aldosterone system (RAAS) with subsequent fibrosis and inflammation [27, 28]. Deregulation of oxidant enzymes is associated with inactivation of ROS scavengers including superoxide dismutase, catalase, metallothionein, and glutathione peroxidase. Enhanced ROS generation also elicits inflammatory and pro-apoptotic transcriptional programs via activation of a molecular complex known as Forkhead box "O" (FOXO) [29]. Inactivation of sirtuins (SIRT1) in the diabetic heart favors FOXO acetylation and subsequent expression of genes favoring cellular apoptosis, cell cycle arrest, accumulation of ROS as well as metabolic derangements [30]. Taken together, increase in circulating FFAs lead to impaired insulin signaling, decreased glucose oxidation, and subsequent hyperglycemia. These events are able to derail pathways leading to myocardial fibrosis, contractile dysfunction, inflammation, mitochondrial insufficiency, and apoptosis (Fig. 5.3).

References

1. Kannel WB, McGee DL (1979) Diabetes and cardiovascular disease. The Framingham study. JAMA 241:2035–2038
2. Shindler DM, Kostis JB, Yusuf S, Quinones MA, Pitt B, Stewart D et al (1996) Diabetes mellitus, a predictor of morbidity and mortality in the Studies of Left Ventricular Dysfunction (SOLVD) Trials and Registry. Am J Cardiol 77:1017–1020

3. Ryden L, Armstrong PW, Cleland JG, Horowitz JD, Massie BM, Packer M et al (2000) Efficacy and safety of high-dose lisinopril in chronic heart failure patients at high cardiovascular risk, including those with diabetes mellitus. Results from the ATLAS trial. Eur Heart J 21:1967–1978

4. Ghose JC, Chakraborty S, Mondal M, Bhandari B (1993) Effect of vasodilator therapy on mortality in chronic congestive heart failure. J Assoc Physicians India 41:269–271

5. Ingelsson E, Sundstrom J, Arnlov J, Zethelius B, Lind L (2005) Insulin resistance and risk of congestive heart failure. JAMA 294:334–341

6. Hofsten DE, Logstrup BB, Moller JE, Pellikka PA, Egstrup K (2009) Abnormal glucose metabolism in acute myocardial infarction: influence on left ventricular function and prognosis. JACC Cardiovasc Imaging 2:592–599

7. Hardin NJ (1996) The myocardial and vascular pathology of diabetic cardiomyopathy. Coron Artery Dis 7:99–108

8. Bugger H, Bode C (2015) The vulnerable myocardium. Diabetic cardiomyopathy. Hamostaseologie 35:17–24

9. Pappachan JM, Varughese GI, Sriraman R, Arunagirinathan G (2013) Diabetic cardiomyopathy: pathophysiology, diagnostic evaluation and management. World J Diabetes 4:177–189

10. Teupe C, Rosak C (2012) Diabetic cardiomyopathy and diastolic heart failure – difficulties with relaxation. Diabetes Res Clin Pract 97: 185–194

11. Owan TE, Hodge DO, Herges RM, Jacobsen SJ, Roger VL, Redfield MM (2006) Trends in prevalence and outcome of heart failure with preserved ejection fraction. N Engl J Med 355:251–259

12. Falcao-Pires I, Leite-Moreira AF (2012) Diabetic cardiomyopathy: understanding the molecular and cellular basis to progress in diagnosis and treatment. Heart Fail Rev 17:325–344

13. Ng AC, Delgado V, Bertini M, van der Meer RW, Rijzewijk LJ, Hooi Ewe S et al (2010) Myocardial steatosis and biventricular strain and strain rate imaging in patients with type 2 diabetes mellitus. Circulation 122:2538–2544

14. Ussher JR (2014) The role of cardiac lipotoxicity in the pathogenesis of diabetic cardiomyopathy. Expert Rev Cardiovasc Ther 12:345–358

15. van de Weijer T, Schrauwen-Hinderling VB, Schrauwen P (2011) Lipotoxicity in type 2 diabetic cardiomyopathy. Cardiovasc Res 92: 10–18

16. Schilling JD, Mann DL (2012) Diabetic cardiomyopathy: bench to bedside. Heart Fail Clin 8:619–631

17. Lee TI, Kao YH, Chen YC, Huang JH, Hsiao FC, Chen YJ (2013) Peroxisome proliferator-activated receptors modulate cardiac dysfunction in diabetic cardiomyopathy. Diabetes Res Clin Pract 100:330–339

18. Finck BN, Han X, Courtois M, Aimond F, Nerbonne JM, Kovacs A et al (2003) A critical role for PPARalpha-mediated lipotoxicity in the pathogenesis of diabetic cardiomyopathy: modulation by dietary fat content. Proc Natl Acad Sci U S A 100:1226–1231

19. Ilkun O, Boudina S (2013) Cardiac dysfunction and oxidative stress in the metabolic syndrome: an update on antioxidant therapies. Curr Pharm Des 19:4806–4817

20. Connelly KA, Kelly DJ, Zhang Y, Prior DL, Advani A, Cox AJ et al (2009) Inhibition of protein kinase C-beta by ruboxistaurin preserves cardiac function and reduces extracellular matrix production in diabetic cardiomyopathy. Circ Heart Fail 2:129–137

21. Giles TD, Ouyang J, Kerut EK, Given MB, Allen GE, McIlwain EF et al (1998) Changes in protein kinase C in early cardiomyopathy and in gracilis muscle in the BB/Wor diabetic rat. Am J Physiol 274: H295–H307

22. Li Z, Abdullah CS, Jin ZQ (2014) Inhibition of PKC-theta preserves cardiac function and reduces fibrosis in streptozotocin-induced diabetic cardiomyopathy. Br J Pharmacol 171:2913–2924

23. Soetikno V, Sari FR, Sukumaran V, Lakshmanan AP, Mito S, Harima M et al (2012) Curcumin prevents diabetic cardiomyopathy in streptozotocin-induced diabetic rats: possible involvement of PKC-MAPK signaling pathway. Eur J Pharm Sci 47:604–614

24. Wakasaki H, Koya D, Schoen FJ, Jirousek MR, Ways DK, Hoit BD et al (1997) Targeted overexpression of protein kinase C beta2 isoform in myocardium causes cardiomyopathy. Proc Natl Acad Sci U S A 94:9320–9325

25. Cai L, Kang YJ (2001) Oxidative stress and diabetic cardiomyopathy: a brief review. Cardiovasc Toxicol 1:181–193

26. Chiu J, Farhangkhoee H, Xu BY, Chen S, George B, Chakrabarti S (2008) PARP mediates structural alterations in diabetic cardiomyopathy. J Mol Cell Cardiol 45:385–393

27. Acar E, Ural D, Bildirici U, Sahin T, Yilmaz I (2011) Diabetic cardiomyopathy. Anadolu Kardiyol Derg 11:732–737

28. Dong B, Yu QT, Dai HY, Gao YY, Zhou ZL, Zhang L et al (2012) Angiotensin-converting enzyme-2 overexpression improves left ventricular remodeling and function in a rat model of diabetic cardiomyopathy. J Am Coll Cardiol 59:739–747

29. Battiprolu PK, Hojayev B, Jiang N, Wang ZV, Luo X, Iglewski M et al
    (2012) Metabolic stress-induced activation of FoxO1 triggers diabetic
    cardiomyopathy in mice. J Clin Invest 122:1109–1118
30. Sulaiman M, Matta MJ, Sunderesan NR, Gupta MP, Periasamy M,
    Gupta M (2010) Resveratrol, an activator of SIRT1, upregulates sarco-
    plasmic calcium ATPase and improves cardiac function in diabetic
    cardiomyopathy. Am J Physiol Heart Circ Physiol 298:H833–H843

Chapter 6
Cerebrovascular Disease

6.1 Prevalence and Prognosis of Cerebrovascular Disease in Diabetic Patients

Ischemic cerebrovascular disease causes approximately 700,000 deaths/year only in the USA with the subtypes of ischemic stroke and transient ischemic attack (TIA) being the most common events (80–85 %) [1–4]. Ischemic stroke remains a very high risk condition which in most of cases does not receive adequate treatment. Many patients presenting at the emergency department have hyperglycemia which may be the result of acute ischemia and altered glucose homeostasis [5, 6]. Hyperglycemia may significantly affect prognosis in these patients [7]. This notion is confirmed by the fact that patients with DM have a 2–4 higher risk of cerebrovascular disease as compared with the non-DM counterpart [8]. Population based studies have shown that DM is an independent risk factor for stroke, with hazard rations of 1.8 in men and 2.2 in women aged 50–79 years [9]. A recent meta-analysis including more than 530,000 subjects demonstrated that patients with DM had a 2.3 relative risk for ischemic stroke as compared with non-DM

F. Paneni, F. Cosentino, *Diabetes and Cardiovascular Disease:*   59
A Guide to Clinical Management, DOI 10.1007/978-3-319-17762-5_6,
© Springer International Publishing Switzerland 2015

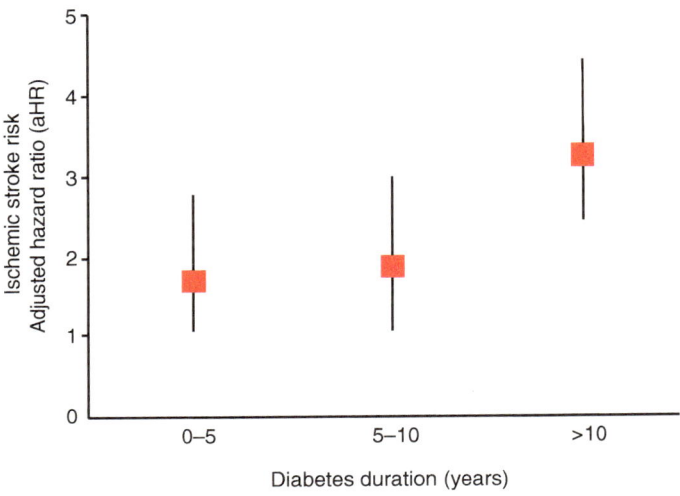

Fig. 6.1 Diabetes duration and risk of stroke. Data from Banerjee et al. [1]

individuals [10]. Noteworthy, the duration of DM is a predictor
of ischemic stroke, even after adjustment for concomitant risk
factors [1]. Patients with DM duration >10 years display a 3.2
relative risk whereas hazard ratio is 1.7 when disease duration is
<5 years (Fig. 6.1) [1]. Moreover, stroke risk is strongly related
to poor glycemic control. Indeed, observational studies show a
linear relationship between HbA_{1c} and the risk of stroke [11].
The occurrence of stroke in patients with DM is explained by
atherosclerotic disease of intracranial and extracranial vessels
[12]. Moreover, a consistent proportion of DM patients suffer
from cardioembolic stroke, which is mostly due to atrial fibrillation and cardiomyopathy. DM increases the risk of all subtypes of stroke: lacunar, large artery occlusive, and
thromboembolic [13]. The latter is the one associated with
larger infarct size and worse prognosis [8].

6.2 Pathophysiology

Understanding the link between hyperglycemia and cerebrovascular disease is of paramount importance for the development of mechanisms-based therapeutic strategies in this setting. In experimental models of ischemic stroke, hyperglycemia is associated with irreversible neuronal damage, intracellular acidosis, delayed NADH regeneration, as well as increased infarct size [7, 14]. Interestingly, the extension of the ischemic damage is directly related to the hyperglycemic burden [15, 16]. High glucose levels may also affect the reperfusion phase by altering the properties of neuronal and vascular cells. Specifically, vascular permeability is increased in diabetic animals, and this phenomenon accounts for increased edema and worse prognosis [16]. Such defects can be explained by maladaptive signaling pathways affecting NO bioavailability, vascular tone, and permeability [17]. Several mechanisms are implicated in hyperglycemia-induced cerebrovascular damage (Fig. 6.2). The hyperglycemic environment activates PKC in cerebral vessels leading to ROS generation, NO degradation, and increased vascular tone. Selective inhibition of PKCδ isoform significantly reduces cerebral infarct size, suggesting that targeting this enzyme may represent a potential approach to combat cerebral microvascular disease in patients with DM [18]. The Rho kinase pathways also contributes to alter the vascular phenotype in this setting [19]. Once activated, such kinase drives a profound rearrangement in the cytoskeleton of vascular smooth muscle cells (VSMSc) thus increasing vascular tone in the brain of diabetic animals. Although it is well established that Rho kinase contributes to vascular damage in the diabetic brain, the link between hyperglycemia and kinase activation remains to be fully elucidated. Changes in vascular tone due to impaired NO delivery and cytoskeletal abnormalities are associated with pro-inflammatory events of the arterial wall favoring a pathological remodeling of

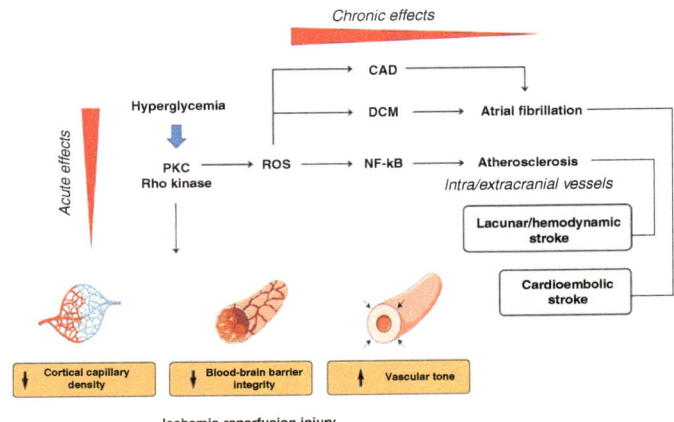

Fig. 6.2 Acute and chronic effects of hyperglycemia in the pathogenesis of ischemic stroke. *CAD* coronary artery disease, *DCM* diabetic cardiomyopathy, *PKC* protein kinase C, *NF-kB* nuclear factor kappa-B, *ROS* reactive oxygen species

the vascular bed characterized by perivascular fibrosis, blood brain barrier permeability, thickening of capillary basal membrane as well as reduced capillary density. Alterations of tight junction proteins OCLN and ZO-1 are also involved in increased vascular permeability [20]. In this regard, experimental evidence suggest that hyperglycemia causes increased matrix metalloproteinase (MMP) activity with subsequent loss of tight junction proteins, thus affecting blood brain barrier integrity [20].

6.3   Clinical Evidence

Preclinical studies confirmed that such structural and functional alterations are also found in patients with DM [21]. In T2D subjects, SPECT analysis has shown that a poor metabolic control significantly correlates with defects in cerebral perfusion, inflammation, and oxidative stress [22]. By contrast, these parameters were improved by an intensive glycemic control, thus strengthening the importance of hyperglycemia in this setting. A meta-analysis has demonstrated that 30-day mortality is significantly higher in DM patients presenting with marked hyperglycemia during ischemic stroke [10]. Based on these observations, several randomized studies were launched to test whether treating acute hyperglycemia may reduce mortality in patients with stroke. In the GIST-UK study, non-DM patients with acute hyperglycemia were treated intravenously (iv) with insulin-glucose-potassium infusion during the first 24 h from the event [23]. This study did not show any benefit despite an adequate metabolic control in the acute phase. Similarly, the THIS trial has reported that intensive glycemic control failed to reduce short-term morbidity and mortality in DM patients with ischemic stroke [24]. Although glycemic control represents a cornerstone in DM treatment, hyperglycemia alone may not explain the increased mortality risk in patients with cerebral ischemia. An accurate control of other risk factors clustering with hyperglycemia is warranted to significantly reduce CV risk in primary and secondary prevention.

References

1. Banerjee C, Moon YP, Paik MC, Rundek T, Mora-McLaughlin C, Vieira JR et al (2012) Duration of diabetes and risk of ischemic stroke: the Northern Manhattan Study. Stroke 43:1212–1217
2. Air EL, Kissela BM (2007) Diabetes, the metabolic syndrome, and ischemic stroke: epidemiology and possible mechanisms. Diabetes Care 30:3131–3140
3. Hewitt J, Castilla Guerra L, Fernandez-Moreno Mdel C, Sierra C (2012) Diabetes and stroke prevention: a review. Stroke Res Treat 2012:673187
4. Meschia JF, Bushnell C, Boden-Albala B, Braun LT, Bravata DM, Chaturvedi S et al (2014) Guidelines for the primary prevention of

stroke: a statement for healthcare professionals from the American Heart Association/American Stroke Association. Stroke 45:3754–3832

5. Lei C, Wu B, Liu M, Chen Y (2015) Association between hemoglobin A1C levels and clinical outcome in ischemic stroke patients with or without diabetes. J Clin Neurosci 22:498–503

6. Luitse MJ, Biessels GJ, Rutten GE, Kappelle LJ (2012) Diabetes, hyperglycaemia, and acute ischaemic stroke. Lancet Neurol 11:261–271

7. Baird TA, Parsons MW, Barber PA, Butcher KS, Desmond PM, Tress BM et al (2002) The influence of diabetes mellitus and hyperglycaemia on stroke incidence and outcome. J Clin Neurosci 9:618–626

8. Hill MD (2014) Stroke and diabetes mellitus. Handb Clin Neurol 126:167–174

9. Barrett-Connor E, Khaw KT (1988) Diabetes mellitus: an independent risk factor for stroke? Am J Epidemiol 128:116–123

10. Sarwar N, Gao P, Seshasai SR, Gobin R, Kaptoge S, Di Angelantonio E et al (2010) Diabetes mellitus, fasting blood glucose concentration, and risk of vascular disease: a collaborative meta-analysis of 102 prospective studies. Lancet 375:2215–2222

11. Di Angelantonio E, Gao P, Khan H, Butterworth AS, Wormser D, Kaptoge S et al (2014) Glycated hemoglobin measurement and prediction of cardiovascular disease. JAMA 311:1225–1233

12. Ergul A, Kelly-Cobbs A, Abdalla M, Fagan SC (2012) Cerebrovascular complications of diabetes: focus on stroke. Endocr Metab Immune Disord Drug Targets 12:148–158

13. Baliga BS, Weinberger J (2006) Diabetes and stroke: part one – risk factors and pathophysiology. Curr Cardiol Rep 8:23–28

14. Elgebaly MM, Ogbi S, Li W, Mezzetti EM, Prakash R, Johnson MH et al (2011) Neurovascular injury in acute hyperglycemia and diabetes: a comparative analysis in experimental stroke. Transl Stroke Res 2:391–398

15. Pulsinelli WA, Levy DE, Sigsbee B, Scherer P, Plum F (1983) Increased damage after ischemic stroke in patients with hyperglycemia with or without established diabetes mellitus. Am J Med 74:540–544

16. Ergul A, Li W, Elgebaly MM, Bruno A, Fagan SC (2009) Hyperglycemia, diabetes and stroke: focus on the cerebrovasculature. Vascul Pharmacol 51:44–49

17. Martini SR, Kent TA (2007) Hyperglycemia in acute ischemic stroke: a vascular perspective. J Cereb Blood Flow Metab 27:435–451

18. Bright R, Steinberg GK, Mochly-Rosen D (2007) DeltaPKC mediates microcerebrovascular dysfunction in acute ischemia and in chronic hypertensive stress in vivo. Brain Res 1144:146–155

19. Chrissobolis S, Sobey CG (2006) Recent evidence for an involvement of rho-kinase in cerebral vascular disease. Stroke 37:2174–2180

20. Hawkins BT, Lundeen TF, Norwood KM, Brooks HL, Egleton RD (2007) Increased blood-brain barrier permeability and altered tight junctions in experimental diabetes in the rat: contribution of hyperglycaemia and matrix metalloproteinases. Diabetologia 50:202–211

21. Clark ME, Payton JE, Pittiglio LI (2014) Acute ischemic stroke and hyperglycemia. Crit Care Nurs Q 37:182–187

22. Cosentino F, Battista R, Scuteri A, De Sensi F, De Siati L, Di Russo C et al (2009) Impact of fasting glycemia and regional cerebral perfusion in diabetic subjects: a study with technetium-99 m-ethyl cysteinate dimer single photon emission computed tomography. Stroke 40:306–308

23. Gray CS, Hildreth AJ, Sandercock PA, O'Connell JE, Johnston DE, Cartlidge NE et al (2007) Glucose-potassium-insulin infusions in the management of post-stroke hyperglycaemia: the UK Glucose Insulin in Stroke Trial (GIST-UK). Lancet Neurol 6:397–406

24. Bruno A, Kent TA, Coull BM, Shankar RR, Saha C, Becker KJ et al (2008) Treatment of hyperglycemia in ischemic stroke (THIS): a randomized pilot trial. Stroke 39:384–389

Part II
Management of Cardiovascular Risk Factors

Chapter 7
Risk Stratification

7.1 Risk Engines

Although considerable efforts in developing effective therapeutic tools, stratification of CV risk in patients with DM remains a major challenge [1, 2]. The issue of risk stratification deserves attention because not every DM subject carries the same degree of inflammation and oxidative stress. The diversity of metabolic phenotypes with different outcomes underscores the need for novel approaches to be used within such heterogeneous population [3]. The easiest and cost-effective tool to estimate risk of CV events is represented by common risk calculators, which are based on the information provided by seminal prospective international registries [4]. Once all risk factors have been identified, CV risk charts or calculator should be used to estimate the total risk of developing CVD over the following 10 years. A total CVD risk of > 20 % in 10 years is defined as high risk. People with moderate-to-high risk are more likely to be compliant with lifestyle changes and preventative medication if given information about their individual CV risk. One of the most powerful calculator (90 % sensitivity) is the UKPDS, a

T2D-specific risk calculator based on 53,000 patient-years of data from the UK Prospective Diabetes Study [5, 6]. The UKPDS Risk Engine provides risk estimates and 95 % confidence intervals, in individuals with T2D not known to have heart disease. This risk engine provides information on the risk of nonfatal and fatal coronary heart disease as well as nonfatal and fatal stroke. These can be calculated for any given duration of T2D based on current age, gender, ethnicity, smoking status, presence or absence of atrial fibrillation, and levels of HbA_{1c}, systolic blood pressure, total cholesterol, and HDL cholesterol (Fig. 7.1) [7]. More recently, the ADVANCE (*Action in Diabetes and Vascular Disease: Preterax and Diamicron Modified Release Controlled Evaluation*) has emerged as an alternative model for CV risk prediction [8]. This model, which incorporates age at diagnosis, known duration of DM, sex, pulse pressure, treated hypertension, atrial fibrillation, retinopathy, HbA_{1c}, urinary albumin/creatinine ratio, and non-HDL cholesterol at baseline, displayed an acceptable discrimination and good calibration during internal validation. A recent meta-analysis testing the predictive performance of CV risk scores found that reliability may vary substantially according to the different populations studied [9]. Interestingly, this study demonstrated that risk scores developed in individuals with DM seemed to estimate CV risk more accurately than those developed in the general population.

7.2   Application of Risk Calculators

An important consideration is that risk charts should be used only in DM patient without evidence of atherosclerotic vascular disease or relevant comorbidities [10]. This is because formal risk assessment is not necessary in those DM patients considered already to be at high enough risk to justify lifestyle and other interventions (antithrombotic, antihypertensive, and

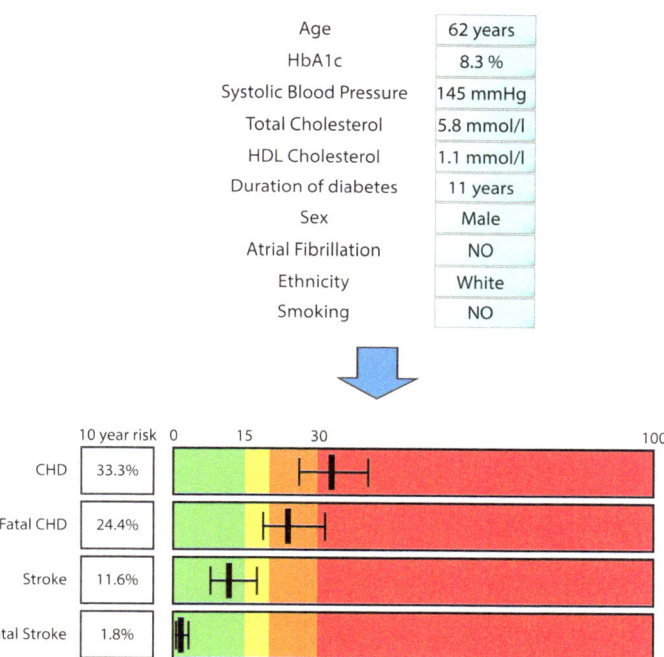

Fig. 7.1 The UKPDS Risk Engine provides risk estimates and 95 % confidence intervals, in individuals with T2D not known to have heart disease, for: nonfatal and fatal coronary heart disease as well as nonfatal and fatal stroke. These can be calculated for any given duration of T2D based on current age, sex, ethnicity, smoking status, presence or absence of atrial fibrillation, and levels of HbA$_{1c}$, systolic blood pressure, total cholesterol and HDL cholesterol

lipid-lowering therapies). For instance it is not useful to stratify CV risk in T2D patients with the following conditions:

- Hypertension ($\geq$160/100 mmHg) with target organ damage
- Evidence of atherosclerotic CVD
- Renal dysfunction (including diabetic nephropathy)
- Severe hypercholesterolemia or inherited dyslipidemias
- People aged 75 or older

Table 7.1 Diagnostic accuracy of established and emerging markers for the prediction of cardiovascular risk in patients with diabetes

Indicators of increased CV risk	Diagnostic accuracy
Established markers	
Microalbuminuria (30–300 mg/24 h), or albumin-creatinine ratio (30–300 mg/g; 3.4–34 mg/mmol)	+++
Carotid wall thickening (IMT >0.9 mm) or plaque	+++
Carotid-femoral PWV >10 m/s	++
Ankle-brachial index <0.9	++
Pulse pressure ≥60 mmHg	++
CKD with eGFR 30–60 ml/min/1.73 m^2 (BSA)	+++
Electrocardiographic LVH (Sokolow-Lyon index >3.5 mV; RaVL >1.1 mV; Cornell voltage duration product >244 mV*ms)	+++
Echocardiographic LVH [LVM index: men >115 g/m^2; women >95 g/m^2 (BSA)]	+++
Emerging markers	
CT scan coronary artery calcium (CAC)	++
C-reactive protein	+
Advanced glycation end products (MG-H1, CML)	++
DNA methylation	+
Inflammatory cytokines IL-1β and IL-6	+
Circulating microRNAs (miR-126)	+
Myeloid calcifying cells (MCCs)	+

CIMT carotid intima-media thickness, *PWV* pulse-wave velocity, *CKD* chronic kidney disease, *BSA* body surface area, *LVH* left ventricular hypertrophy

7.3   Biomarkers

Our understanding of the mechanisms involved in diabetic vascular complications may be instrumental to identify potential biochemical precursors of CV damage in DM (Table 7.1). The *Atherosclerotic Risk in Communities* (ARIC) study prospectively evaluated whether adding C-reactive protein or 18 other novel risk factors individually to a basic risk model would improve prediction of incident CAD in middle-aged men and women [11]. Unfortunately, none of these risk markers predicted CVD beyond established risk calculators. Beside these disappointing results, current ESC/EASD guidelines confirm that albuminuria remains the most powerful predictor of incident CV events and heart failure in T2D patients and recommend to estimate urinary albumin excretion rate when performing risk stratification in DM subjects [10, 12, 13]. Moreover, commonly used vascular risk calculators may be flawed and clinicians are aware of their important variability and limitations [9].

7.3.1 DNA Methylation

The clinical utility of genetic biomarkers for prediction and prevention of CAD has proved to be limited [14]. Recent evidence suggest that epigenetics might better satisfy the unmet needs in CVD prevention. DNA methylation is a well-established mechanism regulating gene transcription [15]. Reduced promoter methylation has been linked to upregulation of genes involved in inflammation, adiposity, beta cell dysfunction, and oxidative vascular damage [16, 17]. Patients with the metabolic syndrome (MS) display relative DNA hypomethylation as compared to those without MS [18]. In this study, fasting plasma glucose and high-density lipoprotein cholesterol were the main MS features associated with DNA hypomethylation. Furthermore, in the same study people with T2D or impaired glucose tolerance had DNA hypomethylation as compared to normoglycemic individuals. The possibility that modification of the epigenome may help to predict vascular risk will be strongly supported by large-scale initiatives such as the *International Human Epigenome Consortium*, aimed at mapping 1,000 reference epigenomes within a decade [19]. Such wide epigenomic analysis will be instrumental for the identification of epigenetic variations specifically associated with major pathological states including T2D and CVD. Together with epigenomics, the predictive value of other high-throughput "omics" technologies such as metabolomics, transcriptomics, and proteomics are being intensively studied in T2D patients, with the aim to obtain large-scale snapshots of the etiological processes linking DM and vascular disease.

7.3.2   MicroRNAs

MicroRNAs (miRs), a newly identified class of small noncoding RNAs, are emerging as key players in the pathogenesis of vascular damage in DM [20]. These small noncoding RNAs regulate gene expression at the post-transcriptional level. Microarray profiling has shown altered miRs expression in subjects with T2D [21]. In this study, T2D patients had a significant deregulation of miRs involved in angiogenesis, vascular repair, and endothelial homeostasis. Among other miRs, miR-126, an important pro-angiogenic effector, was significantly downregulated in plasma samples of 822 patients from the Brunick cohort. Similarly, expression analysis of miR-126 in circulating microparticles from 176 patients with stable CAD with and without DM revealed a significantly reduced miR-126 expression in microparticles from DM patients [22].

7.3.3   Inflammatory Cytokines

Inflammation represents a key fingerprint of metabolic disease. A case-control study within the prospective population-based EPIC (*European Prospective Investigation into Cancer and Nutrition*) study has demonstrated that a combined elevation of

IL-1β and IL-6 was independently associated with an increased risk of T2D, suggesting the importance of low-grade inflammation in the pathogenesis of DM [23]. Another study showed that IL-6 is significantly increased in DM patients undergoing PCI with peri-interventional hyperglycemic state and inversely correlates with responsiveness to clopidogrel and aspirin [24]. By contrast, other indices of systemic inflammation such as C-reactive protein failed to predict incident CVD in DM subjects [3].

7.3.4 Vascular Calcification Markers

Vascular calcification is a pathological hallmark of atherosclerosis in DM subjects [25, 26]. Recent work has suggested that excess concentration of procalcific factors as well as reduction of osteogenic inhibitors may be involved in this process [26]. Circulating osteoblastic cells isolated from human peripheral blood are able to calcify in vitro and in vivo. These cells, which express the bone protein osteocalcin (OC) and bone alkaline phosphatase (BAP), have been considered circulating osteoprogenitor cells and might participate to vascular calcification and atherosclerosis [27]. Indeed, preliminary clinical studies found that coronary atherosclerosis and arterial stiffening are associated with activation of an osteogenic program in bone marrow-derived cells [27]. A recent study has identified a subtype of circulating inflammatory monocytes, called myeloid calcifying cells (MCCs), which are involved in vascular calcification and are over-represented in patients with T2D [28]. MCCs have also been reported to exert anti-angiogenic activity, further contributing to the diabetic vascular disease phenotype. Hence, this cell subpopulation may represent an important tool to stratify CV risk in DM [25].

7.3.5 *Advanced Glycation End-Products (AGEs)*

Advanced glycation end-products (AGEs) are a large family of extensively sugar-modified proteins which can be formed in atherosclerotic plaques as a consequence of increased metabolic activity [29]. Measuring AGEs in the skin using auto-fluorescence has provided important information on risk stratification in DM patients. A study involving 972 DM patients demonstrated that the addition of skin AGEs to the UKPDS risk engine resulted in reclassification of 27 % of the patients from the low- to the high-risk group [30]. Indeed, the 10-year CV event rate was higher in patients with a UKPDS score >10 % when skin AGEs were above the median (56 vs. 39 %). A recent work found that two major AGEs, the methylglyoxal-derived 5-hydro-5-methylimidazolone (MG-H1) and Nε (carboxylmethyl)lysine (CML), measured with tandem mass spectrometry, were significantly higher in symptomatic as compared with asymptomatic carotid plaques [31]. MG-H1 and CML were associated with increased levels of inflammatory cytokines IL-8 and MCP-1 as well as with higher activity of MMP-9, suggesting that AGEs may also provide information on plaque composition and stability. The relevance of AGEs is outlined by the notion that blocking their synthesis may rescue pathological features of DM-related vascular dysfunction. Pharmacological AGEs degradation by the cross-link breaker ALT-711 reduced arterial pulse pressure and improved the compliance of large arteries [32]. Another study with benfotiamine prevented both macro- and microvascular endothelial dysfunction and oxidative stress induced by an AGE-rich meal [33]. Based on these studies, AGEs formation may represent an upstream event triggering vascular inflammation, oxidative stress, and eventually plaque instability.

7.4   Role of Vascular Imaging

Despite DM being associated with a significant atherosclerotic burden, the role of vascular imaging in this setting remains poorly defined. However, emerging evidence indicates that novel imaging modalities to detect atherosclerotic disease might be useful to stratify CV risk beyond traditional risk score calculators. Coronary artery calcium imaging has been found superior to established risk factors for predicting silent myocardial ischemia (SMI) and short-term outcome in a small cohort of high-risk DM subjects [34]. More recently, the *Diabetes Heart Study* conducted on a total of 1,123 T2D participants aged 34–86 years, showed that computed tomography scans of coronary artery calcium (CAC) predicted CVD over 7.4 year follow-up, regardless of the Framingham Risk score [35]. These data suggest that calcium score may meaningfully reclassify DM patients, suggesting clinical utility as a risk stratification tool in patients already at increased CVD risk. However, the predictive value of CAC in DM patients at average-low risk remains elusive. Furthermore, CAC is a rather expensive tool which may not be sustainable in developing countries and further evidence is warranted before we may consider this as a large scale approach in primary prevention [36]. The assessment of intima-media thickness by carotid ultrasound (CIMT) remains a powerful tool to detect preclinical atherosclerosis in DM patients. A recent meta-analysis which reviewed cross-sectional studies linking CIMT and cardiometabolic disease showed that T2D is associated with a 0.13 mm increase in CIMT compared with non-DM subjects, whereas in patients with IGT, the increase in CIMT was about one-third of that observed in DM. Such difference in CIMT was interpreted as an early aging feature in T2D subjects, accounting for a 40 % increase in the relative risks of myocardial infarction and stroke [37]. In a prospective study, Bernard and colleagues reported that CIMT provides a similar predictive value for coronary events compared with the Framingham score, and suggested that the combination of these two indexes would significantly improve risk prediction in these patients [38]. Furthermore, statistically significant correlations (range 0.3–0.5) between CIMT and coronary atherosclerosis, the latter based on a coronary angiogram, CAC, or intravascular ultrasound, have been noted. Taken together, CIMT measurement may be considered an effective, noninvasive tool which can assist in identifying people with DM who are at higher risk of developing microvascular and macrovascular complications. Beside CIMT, ankle-brachial index (ABI), arterial stiffness by pulse wave velocity (PWV), and cardiac autonomic neuropathy (CAN) by standard reflex tests may be also considered as useful CV markers, adding predictive value to the usual risk estimate [10].

7.5   Detection of Coronary Artery Disease

The initial evaluation of T2D patients should include a risk chart (UKPDS, Framingham, or ADVANCE) and, if risk estimation is not clear enough, this approach should be implemented with established biomarkers (albuminuria) or imaging tests (CIMT, Fig. 7.2). In asymptomatic DM patients at high CV risk, it is advisable to proceed with specific tests for the detection of CAD such as ECG stress test, myocardial scintigraphy, or stress echocardiography. Silent myocardial ischemia (SMI) affects 20–35 % of DM patients who have additional risk factors, and 35–70 % of patients with SMI have significant coronary stenoses on angiography, whereas in the others, SMI may result from coronary microvascular dysfunction. SMI, especially when associated with coronary stenosis, has a relevant predictive value if added to routine risk estimate [39]. The main concern raised by current guidelines is that in asymptomatic patients, routine screening

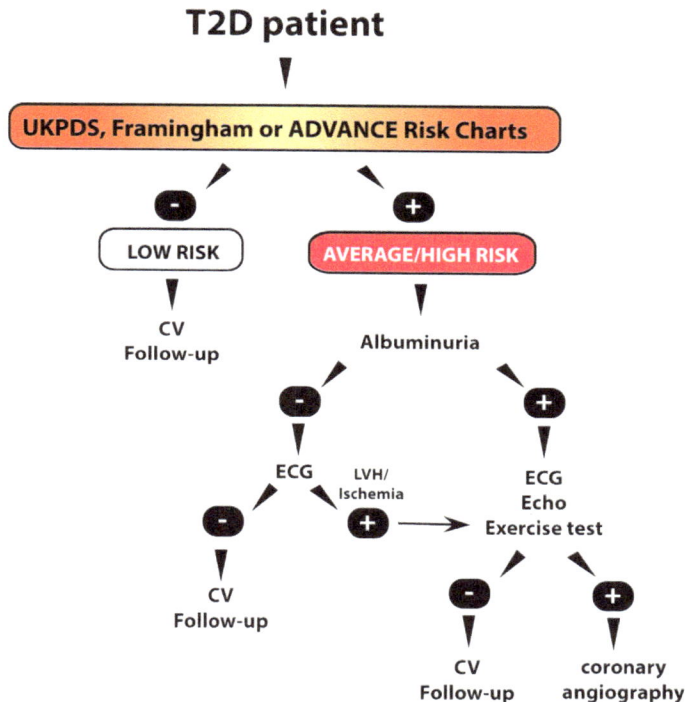

Fig. 7.2 Tentative algorithm for cardiovascular risk stratification in patients with diabetes. *CV* cardiovascular, *LVH* left ventricular hypertrophy, *ECG* electrocardiogram, *Echo* echocardiogram

for CAD is controversial. This is because the benefits of myocardial revascularization in asymptomatic patients remain to be determined. Moreover, it is not clear whether information on the severity of CAD as well as quantification of the ischemic myocardium, as assessed by myocardial scintigraphy, may significantly affect the natural history of CAD. The 5-year follow-up of the DIAD study (*Detection of Ischemia in Asymptomatic Diabetics*) found that SPECT MPI provides good risk stratification, with a sixfold higher risk of cardiac death/nonfatal MI in patients with moderate to large defects versus no or small defects (2.4 % vs. 0.4 %, $p = 0.001$) [40]. However, it does not appear that this information leads to improved clinical care because there was no significant decrease in cardiac death/non-fatal MI in asymptomatic DM individuals screened for ischemia versus routine clinical care. By contrast, data from two large observational cohorts including 11,453 patients (2,206 of whom were diabetic) showed that patients with significant myocardial ischemia on SPECT MPI have improved survival with revascu-larization versus medical therapy in both symptomatic and asymptomatic DM patients [41]. Evidence discussed so far hints that assessment of long-term CV risk may be sufficient to implement intensive therapeutic regimens for the primary prevention of CVD. Further randomized studies are needed to understand whether screening for CAD should be performed in asymptomatic patients at high risk of CV events.

References

1. Paneni F, Costantino S, Cosentino F (2014) Insulin resistance, diabetes, and cardiovascular risk. Curr Atheroscler Rep 16:419
2. Wong ND (2006) Screening and risk stratification of patients with the metabolic syndrome and diabetes. Expert Rev Cardiovasc Ther 4:181–190
3. Paneni F, Costantino S, Cosentino F (2014) Molecular mechanisms of vascular dysfunction and cardiovascular biomarkers in type 2 diabetes. Cardiovasc Diagn Ther 4:324–332
4. Finkelstein EA, Khavjou OA, Will JC, Farris RP, Prabhu M (2006) Assessing the ability of cardiovascular disease risk calculators to evalu-ate effectiveness of trials and interventions. Expert Rev Pharmacoecon Outcomes Res 6:417–424
5. Stevens RJ, Kothari V, Adler AI, Stratton IM, United Kingdom Prospective Diabetes Study Group (2001) The UKPDS risk engine: a model for the risk of coronary heart disease in Type II diabetes (UKPDS 56). Clin Sci (Lond) 101:671–679

6. Guzder RN, Gatling W, Mullee MA, Mehta RL, Byrne CD (2005) Prognostic value of the Framingham cardiovascular risk equation and the UKPDS risk engine for coronary heart disease in newly diagnosed Type 2 diabetes: results from a United Kingdom study. Diabet Med 22:554–562

7. Protopsaltis ID, Konstantinopoulos PA, Kamaratos AV, Melidonis AI (2004) Comparative study of prognostic value for coronary disease risk between the U.K. prospective diabetes study and Framingham models. Diabetes Care 27:277–278

8. Kengne AP, Patel A, Marre M, Travert F, Lievre M, Zoungas S et al (2011) Contemporary model for cardiovascular risk prediction in people with type 2 diabetes. Eur J Cardiovasc Prev Rehabil 18:393–398

9. Allan GM, Garrison S, McCormack J (2014) Comparison of cardiovascular disease risk calculators. Curr Opin Lipidol 25:254–265

10. Ryden L, Grant PJ, Anker SD, Berne C, Cosentino F, Danchin N et al (2013) ESC guidelines on diabetes, pre-diabetes, and cardiovascular diseases developed in collaboration with the EASD: the Task Force on diabetes, pre-diabetes, and cardiovascular diseases of the European Society of Cardiology (ESC) and developed in collaboration with the European Association for the Study of Diabetes (EASD). Eur Heart J 34:3035–3087

11. Folsom AR, Chambless LE, Ballantyne CM, Coresh J, Heiss G, Wu KK et al (2006) An assessment of incremental coronary risk prediction using C-reactive protein and other novel risk markers: the atherosclerosis risk in communities study. Arch Intern Med 166:1368–1373

12. American Diabetes Association (2014) Standards of medical care in diabetes – 2014. Diabetes Care 37(Suppl 1):S14–S80

13. Freedman BI, Langefeld CD, Lohman KK, Bowden DW, Carr JJ, Rich SS et al (2005) Relationship between albuminuria and cardiovascular disease in Type 2 diabetes. J Am Soc Nephrol 16:2156–2161

14. Di Angelantonio E, Butterworth AS (2012) Clinical utility of genetic variants for cardiovascular risk prediction: a futile exercise or insufficient data? Circ Cardiovasc Genet 5:387–390

15. Handy DE, Castro R, Loscalzo J (2011) Epigenetic modifications: basic mechanisms and role in cardiovascular disease. Circulation 123:2145–2156

16. Abi Khalil C (2014) The emerging role of epigenetics in cardiovascular disease. Ther Adv Chronic Dis 5:178–187

17. Burgio E, Lopomo A, Migliore L (2014) Obesity and diabetes: from genetics to epigenetics. Mol Biol Rep. doi:10.1007/s11033-014-3751-z

18. Luttmer R, Spijkerman AM, Kok RM, Jakobs C, Blom HJ, Serne EH et al (2013) Metabolic syndrome components are associated with DNA hypomethylation. Obes Res Clin Pract 7:e106–e115

19. Abbott A (2010) Project set to map marks on genome. Nature 463:
    596–597
20. Quiat D, Olson EN (2013) MicroRNAs in cardiovascular disease: from
    pathogenesis to prevention and treatment. J Clin Invest 123:11–18
21. Zampetaki A, Kiechl S, Drozdov I, Willeit P, Mayr U, Prokopi M et al
    (2010) Plasma microRNA profiling reveals loss of endothelial miR-126
    and other microRNAs in type 2 diabetes. Circ Res 107:810–817
22. Jansen F, Yang X, Hoelscher M, Cattelan A, Schmitz T, Proebsting S
    et al (2013) Endothelial microparticle-mediated transfer of
    MicroRNA-126 promotes vascular endothelial cell repair via SPRED1
    and is abrogated in glucose-damaged endothelial microparticles.
    Circulation 128:2026–2038
23. Spranger J, Kroke A, Mohlig M, Hoffmann K, Bergmann MM, Ristow
    M et al (2003) Inflammatory cytokines and the risk to develop type 2
    diabetes: results of the prospective population-based European
    Prospective Investigation into Cancer and Nutrition (EPIC)-Potsdam
    Study. Diabetes 52:812–817
24. Geisler T, Mueller K, Aichele S, Bigalke B, Stellos K, Htun P et al
    (2010) Impact of inflammatory state and metabolic control on respon-
    siveness to dual antiplatelet therapy in type 2 diabetics after PCI: prog-
    nostic relevance of residual platelet aggregability in diabetics
    undergoing coronary interventions. Clin Res Cardiol 99:743–752
25. Snell-Bergeon JK, Budoff MJ, Hokanson JE (2013) Vascular calcification
    in diabetes: mechanisms and implications. Curr Diab Rep 13:391–402
26. Eghbali-Fatourechi GZ, Lamsam J, Fraser D, Nagel D, Riggs BL,
    Khosla S (2005) Circulating osteoblast-lineage cells in humans. N Engl
    J Med 352:1959–1966
27. Flammer AJ, Gossl M, Widmer RJ, Reriani M, Lennon R, Loeffler D
    et al (2012) Osteocalcin positive CD133+/CD34-/KDR+ progenitor
    cells as an independent marker for unstable atherosclerosis. Eur Heart
    J 33:2963–2969
28. Fadini GP, Albiero M, Menegazzo L, Boscaro E, Vigili de Kreutzenberg
    S, Agostini C et al (2011) Widespread increase in myeloid calcifying
    cells contributes to ectopic vascular calcification in type 2 diabetes.
    Circ Res 108:1112–1121
29. Jandeleit-Dahm K, Cooper ME (2008) The role of AGEs in cardiovas-
    cular disease. Curr Pharm Des 14:979–986
30. Meerwaldt R, Graaff R, Oomen PH, Links TP, Jager JJ, Alderson NL
    et al (2004) Simple non-invasive assessment of advanced glycation
    endproduct accumulation. Diabetologia 47:1324–1330
31. Hanssen NM, Wouters K, Huijberts MS, Gijbels MJ, Sluimer JC,
    Scheijen JL et al (2014) Higher levels of advanced glycation

endproducts in human carotid atherosclerotic plaques are associated with a rupture-prone phenotype. Eur Heart J 35:1137–1146

32. Kass DA, Shapiro EP, Kawaguchi M, Capriotti AR, Scuteri A, deGroof RC et al (2001) Improved arterial compliance by a novel advanced glycation end-product crosslink breaker. Circulation 104:1464–1470

33. Stirban A, Negrean M, Stratmann B, Gawlowski T, Horstmann T, Gotting C et al (2006) Benfotiamine prevents macro- and microvascular endothelial dysfunction and oxidative stress following a meal rich in advanced glycation end products in individuals with type 2 diabetes. Diabetes Care 29:2064–2071

34. Anand DV, Lim E, Hopkins D, Corder R, Shaw LJ, Sharp P et al (2006) Risk stratification in uncomplicated type 2 diabetes: prospective evaluation of the combined use of coronary artery calcium imaging and selective myocardial perfusion scintigraphy. Eur Heart J 27:713–721

35. Agarwal S, Cox AJ, Herrington DM, Jorgensen NW, Xu J, Freedman BI et al (2013) Coronary calcium score predicts cardiovascular mortality in diabetes: diabetes heart study. Diabetes Care 36:972–977

36. Stefanini GG, Windecker S (2015) Can coronary computed tomography angiography replace invasive angiography? Coronary computed tomography angiography cannot replace invasive angiography. Circulation 131:418–426

37. Gayathri R, Chandni R, Udayabhaskaran V (2012) Carotid artery intima media thickness in relation with atherosclerotic risk factors in patients with type 2 diabetes mellitus. J Assoc Physicians India 60:20–24

38. Bernard S, Serusclat A, Targe F, Charriere S, Roth O, Beaune J et al (2005) Incremental predictive value of carotid ultrasonography in the assessment of coronary risk in a cohort of asymptomatic type 2 diabetic subjects. Diabetes Care 28:1158–1162

39. Valensi P, Lorgis L, Cottin Y (2011) Prevalence, incidence, predictive factors and prognosis of silent myocardial infarction: a review of the literature. Arch Cardiovasc Dis 104:178–188

40. Young LH, Wackers FJ, Chyun DA, Davey JA, Barrett EJ, Taillefer R et al (2009) Cardiac outcomes after screening for asymptomatic coronary artery disease in patients with type 2 diabetes: the DIAD study: a randomized controlled trial. JAMA 301:1547–1555

41. Bourque JM, Beller GA (2011) Stress myocardial perfusion imaging for assessing prognosis: an update. JACC Cardiovasc Imaging 4:1305–1319

Chapter 8
Hyperglycemia

8.1 Glycemic Control and Microvascular Complications

Large randomized studies have established that early intensive metabolic control reduces the risk of DM-related microvascular complications, including diabetic nephropathy, retinopathy, and neuropathy. However, despite compelling outcomes, and the availability of effective therapeutic agents, DM remains a public health burden of epidemic proportion [1]. Long-term follow-up of early intervention studies suggest that the metabolic environment deserves close attention since therein lies a window of opportunity for significantly diminishing and potentially preventing microvascular complications [2]. The landmark *Diabetes Complications and Control Trial* (DCCT) not only demonstrated that intensive glycemic control (goal of HbA_{1c} 6.5 %, mean achieved HbA_{1c} 7 %) in subjects with T1D reduced the risk and progression of microvascular complications compared to conventional therapy but also that even within the intensively treated group, subjects who had DM for several years had a higher incidence of microvascular complications when compared with those with new-onset disease [3]. A clinically relevant observation extrapolated from this study was that the

F. Paneni, F. Cosentino, *Diabetes and Cardiovascular Disease: A Guide to Clinical Management*, DOI 10.1007/978-3-319-17762-5_8, © Springer International Publishing Switzerland 2015

relationship between glucose control (as reflected by the mean on-study HbA_{1c} value) and risk of complications was log-linear and extended down to the normal HbA_{1c} range (<6 %), with no threshold noted [4]. This latter finding strengthens the concept that CV manifestations occur along the "glycemic continuum" and not only within the diabetic condition. The *Epidemiology of Diabetes Interventions and Complications* (EDIC) study, an observational follow-up of DCCT trial, was the first large-scale clinical trial to demonstrate the persistent benefit among patients who were initially randomized to intensive control compared to conventional treatment, despite converging HbA_{1c} values between the two groups [5]. Emerging data from the EDIC also suggest that the influence of early glycemic control on eventual progression of macrovascular complications may become more evident with longer follow-up [6]. Indeed, 9 years after DCCT termination, participants previously randomized to the intensive arm had a 42 % reduction ($p=0.02$) in CVD outcomes and a 57 % reduction ($p=0.02$) in the risk of nonfatal myocardial infarction (MI), stroke, or CVD death compared with those previously in the standard arm [6]. Interestingly, a recent report on the cumulative incidence of diabetic retinopathy after 18-year DCCT follow-up demonstrated that risk of microvascular complications continues to be lower in patients initially randomized to intensive glycemic control, thus strengthening the importance of this approach for the prevention of microvascular outcomes (Fig. 8.1) [7]. Data from the *United Kingdom Prospective Diabetes Study* (UKPDS) appear to be consistent with this evidence. UKPDS, a randomized, prospective, multicenter trial, showed that intensive glucose therapy (median HbA1c 7.0 %) in patients with newly diagnosed T2D was associated with a reduced risk of microvascular complications [8]. In a post-interventional follow-up of the UKPDS survivors performed 10-year later, there was a continued benefit

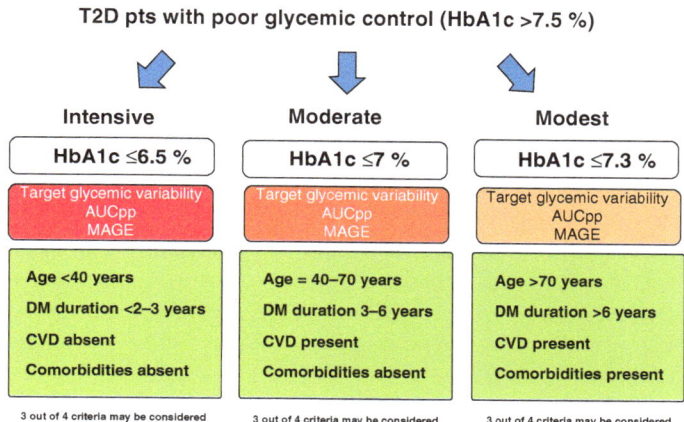

Fig. 8.1 Tentative algorithm for the management of hyperglycemia (HbA$_{1c}$ target) in diabetic patients, according to age, diabetes duration, presence of cardiovascular disease, and comorbidities. Therapeutic strategies to reduce glycemic variability should be also implemented (mostly in young subjects). *CVD* cardiovascular disease, *DM* diabetes, *AUCpp* postprandial incremental area under the curve of blood glucose levels, *MAGE* average glycemic excursions

from the early institution of improved glucose control on micro- and macrovascular outcomes [9]. However, it should be noted that the reduction in CV complications (combined fatal or non-fatal MI, stroke, and sudden death) observed in the intensive glycemic control arm of UKPDS was not statistically significant ($p = 0.052$), and there was no suggestion of benefit on other CVD outcomes such as stroke and peripheral artery disease. Taken together, studies examined so far suggest that intensive glycemic control reduces the risk of microvascular complications whereas its impact on macrovascular disease remains not clearly defined.

8.2   Glycemic Control and Macrovascular Complications

Because of ongoing uncertainty about the effectiveness of intensive glycemic control in reducing DM-related CV events, several large long-term trials were launched in the past decade to compare the effects of intensive versus standard glycemic control on CVD outcomes in relatively high-risk participants with established T2D. The *Action to Control Cardiovascular Risk in Diabetes Study Group* (ACCORD) [10], *Action in Diabetes and Vascular Disease -Preterax and Diamicron Modified Release Controlled Evaluation* (ADVANCE) [11], and the *Veterans Affairs Diabetes Trial* (VADT) [12] sought to determine the effect of glucose lowering to near-normal levels on CV risk. These studies included a large number of participants with complete follow-up for a median of 3.5–5.6 years. The baseline characteristics were typical for adults with T2D: mean age of 60–66 years and duration of DM ranging from 8 to 11 years (Table 8.1). Approximately one-third of patients in each study had a history of CVD, so these trials assessed the effect of intensive glycemic control in patients with and in those without pre-existing atherosclerotic vascular disease. In ADVANCE, microvascular, but not macrovascular complications, were improved during 5-year follow-up. Indeed, intensive glycemic control significantly reduced the primary end point (HR 0.90 [95 % CI 0.82–0.98], $p = 0.01$), but this result was mostly driven by a significant reduction in the microvascular outcome (occurrence of macroalbuminuria, 0.86 [0.77–0.97], $p = 0.01$), with no effects on macrovascular endpoints (0.94 [0.84–1.06], $p = 0.32$). Enthusiasm and hopes of glucose control benefits were struck down by the results of the ACCORD trial, prematurely stopped after 3.4 years due to increased mortality in the intensive treatment arm. Despite many authors having attributed these negative findings to the aggressive control of hyperglycemia, scrutiny

Table 8.1 Main characteristics of recent randomized trials testing the effects of intensive glycemic control on macrovascular complications in high-risk T2D patients

	ACCORD	ADVANCE	VADT
Number of patients	10,251	11,140	1,791
Mean age (years)	62	66	60
Diabetes duration	10	8	11.5
Established CVD (%)	35	32	40
Median HbA$_{1c}$	8.1	7.2	9.4
HbA$_{1c}$ goal (%)	<6	<6.5	<6
Management of other risk factors	Blood pressure and lipids	Blood pressure	Multifactorial treatment
Median follow-up (years)	3.5 (prematurely stopped)	5	5.6
Final HbA$_{1c}$ values	6.4 vs. 7.5	6.3 vs. 7.0	6.9 vs. 8.5
Hypoglycemia			
Intensive arm	16.2	2.7	21.2
Control arm	5.1	1.5	9.9
Definition of primary outcome	Nonfatal MI, nonfatal stroke, CV death	Micro- and macrovascular outcomes	Nonfatal MI, nonfatal stroke, CV death, HF hospitalization, revascularization
HR for primary outcome	0.90 (0.78–1.04)	microvascular: 0.90 (0.82–0.98); macrovascular: 0.94 (0.84–1.06)	0.88 (0.74–1.05)
HR for mortality	1.22 (1.01–1.46)	0.93 (0.83–1.06)	1.07 (0.82–1.42)

CVD cardiovascular disease, *MI* myocardial infarction, *HF* heart failure, *HR* hazard ratio

sub-analyses of the mortality findings in ACCORD (considering variables such as weight gain, use of drug combination, and hypoglycemia) were unable to explain the excess mortality observed in the intensive arm [4]. Yet, glycemic control achieved in the VADT trial had no significant effect on the rates of major CV events, death, or microvascular complications. During a median 5.6-year follow-up period, the cumulative incidence of the primary outcome was not significantly lower in the intensive arm (HR 0.88 [95 % CI 0.74–1.05], $p=0.12$). There were more CVD deaths in the intensive group than in the standard arm (38 vs. 29), but such difference was not statistically significant.

Albeit in all these studies patients were aggressively treated for all other CV risk factors, DM subjects remained exposed to a substantial risk of CV events and mortality [4]. Indeed, a tight control of glycemia together with a multifactorial approach were not able to prevent the development of coronary artery disease in these patients. Possible explanations for these negative results – as previously shown by the DCCT and UKPDS investigators – may be a too short follow-up to demonstrate an effect on macrovascular complications and/or long-standing duration of DM beyond the stage where tight glycemic control could exert any protective effect [4]. Another possible explanation is that in T2D, where other CVD risk factors are highly prevalent, the additive benefits of intensive glycemic control might be difficult to demonstrate. It is likely that a real benefit of glucose lowering on CVD in T2DM, even if it could be proven, is modest compared with and incremental to treatment of other CVD risk factors.

8.3   Hypoglycemia

Intensive glucose lowering increases the incidence of severe hypoglycemia three- to fourfold in both T1D and T2D [13]. The occurrence of hypoglycemia may contribute to explain the failure of intensive glycemic control mostly in the ACCORD and VADT trials where severe hypoglycemia was observed in 16.2 and 21.1 % of patients, respectively (Table 8.1). Post hoc analyses from these trials have shown that hypoglycemia has a detrimental impact on CV morbidity and mortality [14]. Furthermore in the ADVANCE trial patients who experienced severe hypoglycemia were those with the highest mortality after a 5-year follow-up [15]. Severe hypoglycemia was shown to be strongly related to an increased risk of the first macrovascular event (death from a CV cause, nonfatal myocardial infarction, or nonfatal stroke) as well as to higher all-cause, CV and non-CV mortality rates. However, the significance of hypoglycemia is still unclear. Indeed, it is not known whether hypoglycemia per se can affect outcomes in DM patients, via an array of detrimental mechanisms, or, alternatively, whether hypoglycemia is just an epiphenomenon, reflecting the disease severity and the comorbidity burden, simply identifying those at high risk of poor CV outcomes [16]. The latter assumption is supported by the notion that DM patients who are more likely to develop severe hypoglycemic events are older, have lower body mass index, impaired renal function, a history of microvascular complications, dementia, previous hypoglycemic events, longer duration of T2D, and worse education. Moreover, comorbidities may significantly increase the risk of hypoglycemia and this is why glycemic targets should be less stringent in this category of patients. Another precipitating factor is the impaired hypoglycemic awareness which increases with duration of DM and is a significant risk factor for hypoglycemia [17]. The outcome of glucose-lowering studies has raised the question as to whether hypoglycemia is an important risk factor for myocardial infarction in patients with DM. Frier et al. have extensively reviewed this topic, providing evidence for a number of adverse effects of hypoglycemia on the CV system, particularly in the presence of autonomic neuropathy [18].

8.4   Recommended Glycemic Targets

Based on available evidence, recent guidelines on the management of DM do not recommend a very tight glucose control if the ambition is to reduce macrovascular complications [19, 20]. Moreover, in older patients with long-standing DM and CVD, glycemic control should be modest because of a concrete risk of hypoglycemia and other side effects. Intensive glycemic control to achieve a HbA_{1c} target < 7 % is effective but should be applied in an individualized manner taking into account several variables such as (Fig. 8.2):

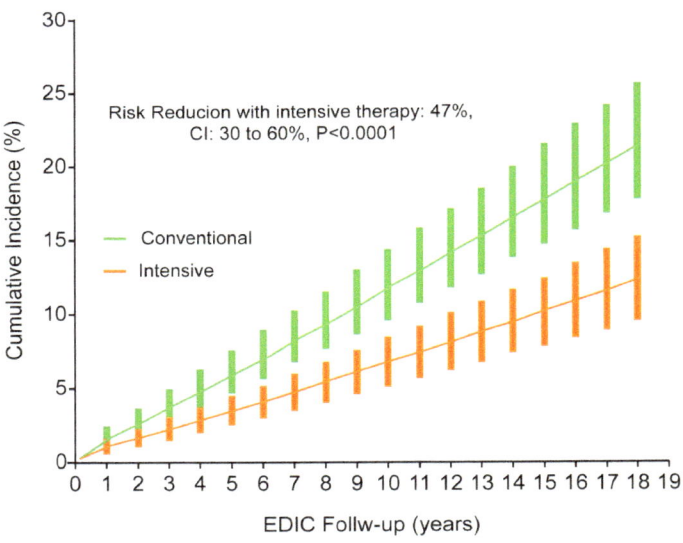

Fig. 8.2 Estimated cumulative incidence of new proliferative diabetic retinopathy during the following 18 years after DCCT termination (Data from The Diabetes Control and Complications Trial (DCCT)/Epidemiology of Diabetes Interventions and Complications (EDIC) Research Group [7])

- Age
- Duration of diabetes
- Presence of cardiovascular disease
- Comorbidities

For the prevention of microvascular complications, HbA_{1c} should be less than 7 %, fasting glycemia <120 mg/dl, and postprandial glycemia <160–180 mg/dl. Postprandial hyperglycemia is a reliable estimate of glycemic variability and it is emerging as a powerful predictor of micro- and macrovascular complications in DM patients, even when adjusted for HbA_{1c} levels. Glycemic variability can be quantified by means of average glycemic excursions (MAGE) and postprandial incremental area under the curve of blood glucose levels (AUCpp) [21]. MAGE have been conceived to measure the mean of the differences between consecutive peaks and nadirs and provide a reliable estimate of glycemic instability. On the other hand, AUCpp is a well-established marker reflecting meal-related hyperglycemic swings. Previous work has shown that postprandial glucose levels are significantly prolonged in T2D patients as compared to healthy controls, and may trigger ROS generation, reduced nitric oxide breakdown, and endothelial damage [22]. Noteworthy, postprandial hyperglycemia is an independent risk factor for vascular complications in T2D [23]. Several studies have demonstrated that in DM patients achieving a HbA_{1c} <6.5 %, glycemic excursions were independently associated to microvascular events [24, 25]. In the ACCORD and ADVANCE trials, the reduction of HbA_{1c} levels was not accompanied by a reduction of glycemic variability and this aspect may have contributed to the lack of CV benefit observed in these trials. In this regard, the STOP-NIDDM trial has shown that decreasing postprandial hyperglycemia is associated with a 49 % relative risk reduction in the development of CV events (HR, 0.51; 95 % confidence interval [CI]; 0.28–0.95; $p = .03$) in high-risk subjects with impaired glucose tolerance [26]. Hence, treatment of hyperglycemia should take into account the suppression of post-prandial hyperglycemia and glycemic excursions which represent important HbA_{1c}-independent markers of cardiovascular risk.

8.5 Cardiovascular Effects of Glucose-Lowering Drugs

Available antidiabetic drugs are effective for the management of hyperglycemia; however many DM patients have cardiovascular problems and attention should be paid to the risk-benefit ration of the different formulations. Adverse CV effects of hypoglycemic agents vary according to mechanism of action and the combination used (Table 8.2). Insulin is widely used to treat hyperglycemia both in T1D and T2D, this drug also protects against postprandial hyperglycemia and may secure glycemic control over 24 h. The ORIGIN trial has recently demonstrated that more than 6 years of treatment with insulin glargine had a neutral effect on CV outcomes and cancers while increased the risk of hypoglycemia and body weight [27]. Sulphonylureas metiglinides and incretin mimetics (GLP-1 analogues and DDP-4 inhibitors) act by stimulating endogen insulin secretion by pancreatic beta cell. Sulphonylureas and metiglinides are associated to increased body weight and hypoglycemia in the absence of clear CV benefits. These drugs may be prescribed to DM patients with CVD but their potential hypoglycemic effects should be strictly monitored by analysis of glycemic profile and blood glucose monitoring, particularly during the first weeks of treatment [28]. GLP-1 and DDP-4 have gastrointestinal side effects and accelerate satiety thus reducing of body weight, an effect which is more pronounced with GLP-1 agonists (Table 8.2). Although these drugs have shown to reduce intermediate and biochemical endpoints such as endothelial function, systemic inflammation, and oxidative stress, recent randomized trials SAVOR-TIMI 53 and EXAMINE did not show any significant benefit on CV outcomes [29]. On the other hand, these drugs did not increase CV risk, suggesting their use as hypoglycemic agents in diabetics with CVD. Pioglitazone, a PPARγ agonist with partial PPARα activity, reduces hyperglycemia by improving peripheral insulin sensitivity and hepatic glucose production, whereas metformin, a biguanide, exerts similar effects by activating the AMP kinase. Pioglitazone has favorable metabolic effects, it improves lipid profile and blood pressure, is associated with low risk of hypoglycemia, and, in the PROActive trial, was associated with a modest CV benefit [28]. However, pioglitazone and rosiglitazione, the latter withdrawn from the market due to increased MI risk, are associated with a number of complications including bladder cancer, bone fractures, fluid retention with increased body weight, and last but not least, risk of heart failure. In order to improve tolerability of these drugs, double PPARαγ agonists have been launched and tested in a large randomized clinical trial. In the AleCardio trial, the use of Aleglitazar was associated with a significant increase of renal and CV complications, leading to a premature interruption of study for safety concerns [30]. As of today, metformin remains the first-line drug for the treatment of T2D [20]. This is because the metformin is well tolerated, reduces body weight, and is associated with reduced risk of nonfatal MI. The inhibitors of glucose intestinal absorption have shown to reduce postprandial hyperglycemia in patients with prediabetes and T2D (Table 8.2) [26]. However, further studies are needed to better characterize the risk-benefit profile of this class of drugs.

Table 8.2 Properties and cardiovascular effects of available glucose-lowering drugs for the treatment of type 2 diabetes

Drugs class	Effect	Hypogly-cemia	Advantages/disadvantages
Metformin	Insulin sensitizer	No	First-line drug for the treatment of T2D
			Reduces risk of MI (UKPDS)
			Several randomized studies available
			Mild side effects
			Cost-effective
Sulphonylureas	Secretagogue	Yes	Several randomized studies available
			Reduces microvascular complications (UKPDS)
			Reduces ischemic *preconditioning*
			Increases the risk of hypoglycemia
			Cost-effective
Meglitinides Repaglinide Nateglinide	Secretagogue	Yes	Weight gain
			Reduce glycemic variability
			Effects on ischemic *preconditioning*
			Increase the risk of hypoglycemia
			High costs
Alpha-glucosidase inhibitors Acarbose Miglitol Voglibose	Inhibit glucose intestinal absorption	No	Further studies needed
			Reduce glycemic variability
			Potential cardiovascular benefit (STOP-NIDDM)
			Frequent gastrointestinal side effects
			Moderate costs

Table 8.2   (continued)

Drugs class	Effect	Hypogly-cemia	Advantages/disadvantages
Thiazolidinediones Pioglitazone Rosiglitazone	Insulin sensitizer	No	Weight gain Reduce risk of MI (PROActive) Improve diabetic dyslipidemia Increase hospitalization for heart failure Increase risk of bladder cancer Bone fractures High costs
GLP-1 agonists Exenatide Liraglutide	Secretagogue	No	Weight gain No reduction of CV endpoints (EXTREME) Improve beta-cell function Gastrointestinal side effects High costs
DPP-4 inhibitors Sitagliptin Saxagliptin Vildagliptin Linagliptin Alogliptin	Secretagogue	No	Well tolerated No reduction of CV endpoints (SAVOR TIMI 53) Modest HbA_{1c} reduction High costs
Insulin	Secretagogue	Yes	Weight gain Reduces glycemic variability Reduces microvascular (UKPDS) but not macrovascular (ORIGIN) complications Increases the risk of hypoglycemia
SGLT2 inhibitors	Inhibit renal transport of glucose	No	Further studies needed High costs

T2D type 2 diabetes, *MI* myocardial infarction

References

1. Fioretto P, Dodson PM, Ziegler D, Rosenson RS (2010) Residual microvascular risk in diabetes: unmet needs and future directions. Nat Rev Endocrinol 6:19–25
2. Ceriello A, Ihnat MA, Thorpe JE (2009) Clinical review 2: the "metabolic memory": is more than just tight glucose control necessary to prevent diabetic complications? J Clin Endocrinol Metab 94:410–415
3. The Diabetes Control and Complications Trial Research Group (1993) The effect of intensive treatment of diabetes on the development and progression of long-term complications in insulin-dependent diabetes mellitus. N Engl J Med 329:977–986
4. Skyler JS, Bergenstal R, Bonow RO, Buse J, Deedwania P, Gale EA et al (2009) Intensive glycemic control and the prevention of cardiovascular events: implications of the ACCORD, ADVANCE, and VA Diabetes Trials: a position statement of the American Diabetes Association and a Scientific Statement of the American College of Cardiology Foundation and the American Heart Association. J Am Coll Cardiol 53:298–304
5. Writing Team for the Diabetes Control, Complications Trial/Epidemiology of Diabetes Interventions, Complications Research Group (2003) Sustained effect of intensive treatment of type 1 diabetes mellitus on development and progression of diabetic nephropathy: the Epidemiology of Diabetes Interventions and Complications (EDIC) study. JAMA 290:2159–2167
6. Nathan DM, Lachin J, Cleary P, Orchard T, Brillon DJ, Backlund JY et al (2003) Intensive diabetes therapy and carotid intima-media thickness in type 1 diabetes mellitus. N Engl J Med 348:2294–2303
7. Diabetes Control Complications Trial/Epidemiology of Diabetes, Interventions Complications Research Group (2015) Effect of intensive diabetes therapy on the progression of diabetic retinopathy in patients with type 1 diabetes: 18 years of follow-up in the DCCT/EDIC. Diabetes 64:631–642
8. UK Prospective Diabetes Study (UKPDS) Group (1998) Intensive blood-glucose control with sulphonylureas or insulin compared with conventional treatment and risk of complications in patients with type 2 diabetes (UKPDS 33). Lancet 352:837–853
9. Holman RR, Paul SK, Bethel MA, Matthews DR, Neil HA (2008) 10-year follow-up of intensive glucose control in type 2 diabetes. N Engl J Med 359:1577–1589
10. Gerstein HC, Miller ME, Byington RP, Goff DC Jr, Bigger JT, Buse JB et al (2008) Effects of intensive glucose lowering in type 2 diabetes. N Engl J Med 358:2545–2559

11. Patel A, MacMahon S, Chalmers J, Neal B, Billot L, Woodward M et al (2008) Intensive blood glucose control and vascular outcomes in patients with type 2 diabetes. N Engl J Med 358:2560–2572

12. Duckworth W, Abraira C, Moritz T, Reda D, Emanuele N, Reaven PD et al (2009) Glucose control and vascular complications in veterans with type 2 diabetes. N Engl J Med 360:129–139

13. Hemmingsen B, Lund SS, Gluud C, Vaag A, Almdal T, Hemmingsen C et al (2011) Intensive glycaemic control for patients with type 2 diabetes: systematic review with meta-analysis and trial sequential analysis of randomised clinical trials. BMJ 343:d6898

14. Goto A, Arah OA, Goto M, Terauchi Y, Noda M (2013) Severe hypoglycaemia and cardiovascular disease: systematic review and meta-analysis with bias analysis. BMJ 347:f4533

15. Zoungas S, Patel A, Chalmers J, de Galan BE, Li Q, Billot L et al (2010) Severe hypoglycemia and risks of vascular events and death. N Engl J Med 363:1410–1418

16. Snell-Bergeon JK, Wadwa RP (2012) Hypoglycemia, diabetes, and cardiovascular disease. Diabetes Technol Ther 14(Suppl 1):S51–S58

17. Ahren B (2013) Avoiding hypoglycemia: a key to success for glucose-lowering therapy in type 2 diabetes. Vasc Health Risk Manag 9: 155–163

18. Frier BM, Schernthaner G, Heller SR (2011) Hypoglycemia and cardiovascular risks. Diabetes Care 34(Suppl 2):S132–S137

19. Ryden L, Grant PJ, Anker SD, Berne C, Cosentino F, Danchin N et al (2013) ESC Guidelines on diabetes, pre-diabetes, and cardiovascular diseases developed in collaboration with the EASD: the Task Force on diabetes, pre-diabetes, and cardiovascular diseases of the European Society of Cardiology (ESC) and developed in collaboration with the European Association for the Study of Diabetes (EASD). Eur Heart J 34:3035–3087

20. American Diabetes Association (2014) Standards of medical care in diabetes – 2014. Diabetes Care 37(Suppl 1):S14–S80

21. Kohnert KD, Heinke P, Vogt L, Salzsieder E (2015) Utility of different glycemic control metrics for optimizing management of diabetes. World J Diabetes 6:17–29

22. Saisho Y (2014) Glycemic variability and oxidative stress: a link between diabetes and cardiovascular disease? Int J Mol Sci 15:18381–18406

23. Cavalot F, Pagliarino A, Valle M, Di Martino L, Bonomo K, Massucco P et al (2011) Postprandial blood glucose predicts cardiovascular events and all-cause mortality in type 2 diabetes in a 14-year follow-up:

lessons from the San Luigi Gonzaga Diabetes Study. Diabetes Care 34:2237–2243

24. Zhang JW, He LJ, Cao SJ, Yang Q, Yang SW, Zhou YJ (2014) Effect of glycemic variability on short term prognosis in acute myocardial infarction subjects undergoing primary percutaneous coronary interventions. Diabetol Metab Syndr 6:76

25. Mi SH, Su G, Li Z, Yang HX, Zheng H, Tao H et al (2012) Comparison of glycemic variability and glycated hemoglobin as risk factors of coronary artery disease in patients with undiagnosed diabetes. Chin Med J 125:38–43

26. Chiasson JL, Josse RG, Gomis R, Hanefeld M, Karasik A, Laakso M et al (2003) Acarbose treatment and the risk of cardiovascular disease and hypertension in patients with impaired glucose tolerance: the STOP-NIDDM trial. JAMA 290:486–494

27. Gerstein HC, Bosch J, Dagenais GR, Diaz R, Jung H, Maggioni AP et al (2012) Basal insulin and cardiovascular and other outcomes in dysglycemia. N Engl J Med 367:319–328

28. Inzucchi SE, Bergenstal RM, Buse JB, Diamant M, Ferrannini E, Nauck M et al (2012) Management of hyperglycemia in type 2 diabetes: a patient-centered approach: position statement of the American Diabetes Association (ADA) and the European Association for the Study of Diabetes (EASD). Diabetes Care 35:1364–1379

29. Paneni F (2014) 2013 ESC/EASD guidelines on the management of diabetes and cardiovascular disease: Established knowledge and evidence gaps. Diab Vasc Dis Res 11:5–10

30. Lincoff AM, Tardif JC, Schwartz GG, Nicholls SJ, Ryden L, Neal B et al (2014) Effect of aleglitazar on cardiovascular outcomes after acute coronary syndrome in patients with type 2 diabetes mellitus: the AleCardio randomized clinical trial. JAMA 311:1515–1525

Chapter 9
Diabetic Dyslipidemia

9.1 Definition and Pathophysiology of Diabetic Dyslipidemia

Insulin resistance in patients with diabetes mellitus (DM) causes metabolic changes by several mechanisms leading to increased levels of small and dense low density lipoprotein cholesterol (sd-LDL-C), low high density lipoprotein cholesterol (HDL-C) and mild or severe hypertriglyceridemia, defining a well-studied phenotype known as atherogenic dyslipidemia [1]. Atherogenic dyslipidemia has been associated with a 3- to 6-fold increase in the risk of CV events [2]. This lipid pattern is a common finding in patients with DM and its prevalence grows with that of visceral obesity [3]. The *European Action on Secondary Prevention through Intervention to Reduce Events* (EUROASPIRE III) survey reported that the overall prevalence of high TG and low HDL–C has almost doubled, compared with the prevalence seen in EUROASPIRE II, due to the increase in T2D and obesity [4, 5]. Adiposity and insulin resistance cause overproduction of VLDL/apolipoprotein B (ApoB) complexes, decreased catabolism of apoB-lipoprotein containing particles, and accelerated degradation of HDL-apoA1. Impaired insulin sensitivity in the adipose tissue significantly

F. Paneni, F. Cosentino, *Diabetes and Cardiovascular Disease:* 101
A Guide to Clinical Management, DOI 10.1007/978-3-319-17762-5_9,
© Springer International Publishing Switzerland 2015

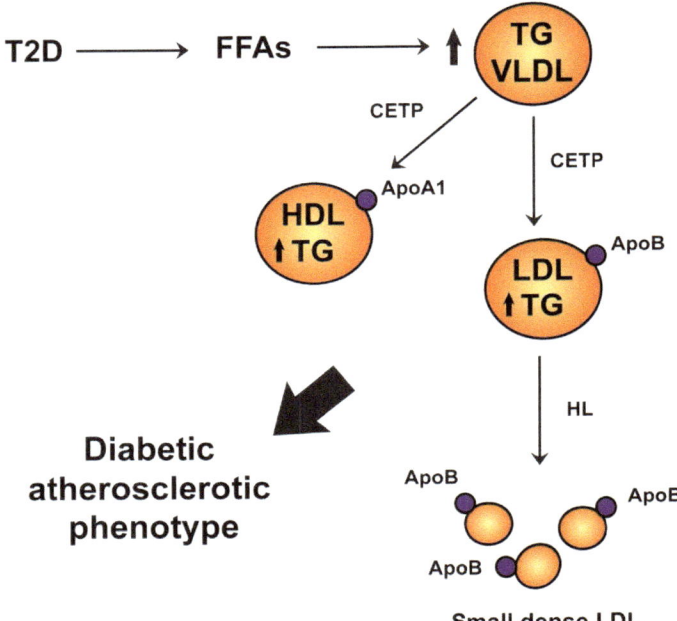

Fig. 9.1 Schematic representation of lipid changes underpinning athero-
genic dyslipidemia in patients with type 2 diabetes. *T2D* type 2 diabetes,
FFAs free fatty acids, *HL* hepatic lipase, *HSL* hormone-sensitive lipase,
IDL intermediate density lipoprotein, *LDL* low density lipoprotein,
HDL-C high density lipoprotein cholesterol, *TG* triglycerides, *VLDL-C*
very low density lipoprotein cholesterol, *apoA1* apolipoprotein A1,
CEPT cholesteryl ester transfer protein

suppresses the inhibition of hormone sensitive lipase (HSL),
thus leading to free fatty acid release (FFA) into the circulation
(Fig. 9.1) [2]. Moreover, hypertrophic adipocytes are defective
in the incorporation of FFA into TG. Such excess of FFA is
subjected to liver reuptake, promoting the synthesis of TG-rich
VLDL-C and apoB [6]. These lipids are substrates for the

cholesterol ester transfer protein (CETP), which transfers TG to LDL-C and HDL-C in exchange for cholesteryl esters. After CETP has transferred TG from VLDL-C to LDL-C, the latter becomes a substrate for the hepatic lipase (HL) whose activity is strongly increased in the presence of insulin resistance (Fig. 9.1). HL-mediated hydrolysis makes LDL-C poor of TG and phospholipids, and this modification leads to smaller LDL which are more prone to oxidation in the vascular wall. This also results in altered ApoB conformation, which weakens its binding to the LDL-C receptor, reduces internalization into the liver and prolongs LDL-C residence time into the circulation [7]. This will increase the chance of sd-LDL to penetrate into the vessel intima where their oxidation promotes vascular inflammation, and atherosclerosis [8].

9.2 LDL Cholesterol Lowering Therapies

Statins remain a cornerstone in the treatment of DM patients and account for the largest reduction of mortality observed in this population [9–11] In the 4S study (*Scandinavian Simvastatin Survival Study*), treatment with simvastatin 20–40 mg significantly reduced the risk of all-cause mortality and myocardial infarction respectively by 43 and 55 % in patients with T2D as compared to 29 and 32 % observed in people without DM [12]. The *Heart Protection Study* has shown that 5-year treatment with simvastatin reduced the CV composite endpoint (acute coronary syndromes, stroke, myocardial revascularization) by 34 %. Similarly, pravastatin 40 mg was associated with a 24 % reduction of CV events in T2D subjects enrolled in the CARE trial (*Cholesterol and Recurrent Events*) [13]. In the 2,532 DM patients enrolled in the ASCOT-LLA study (*Anglo-Scandinavian Cardiac Outcomes Trial-Lipid Lowering Arm*), treatment with atorvastatin led to a 36 % reduction of fatal and nonfatal myocardial infarction after a median follow-up of 3.3 years [14]. Furthermore, in the CARDS trial (*Collaborative Atorvastatin Diabetes Study*) treatment with atorvastatin 10 mg in 2,800 patients with T2D resulted in a 36 % reduction of coronary events, 31 % of revascularization procedures, and decreased the risk of stroke by 48 % [15]. In a meta-analysis of 14 randomized controlled trials including more than 18,000 persons with DM, the mean duration of follow-up was 4.3 years, with 3,247 major vascular events. The study reported a 9 % reduction in all-cause mortality and a 21 % reduction in the incidence of major vascular outcomes per mmol/L of LDL-C lowering (RR 0.79; 99 % Cl 0.72–0.87; $p < 0.0001$), similar to that seen in non-DM. Interestingly, the magnitude of the benefit was associated with the absolute reduction in LDL-C, highlighting a positive relationship between LDL-C and CV risk [16]. Based on the linear relation between LDL cholesterol and CV events, several RCTs tested the hypothesis that higher statin dosages could further reduce CVD burden in DM patients. In diabetics with stable coronary artery disease the TNT trial has shown that atorvastatin 80 mg is able to reduce the occurrence of major CV events as compared to atorvastatin 10 mg [17]. However, data from 10 RCTs, studying 41,778 patients followed for 2.5 years, showed that intensive statin dosage reduced the composite CV endpoint by 10 % (95 % Cl 0.84–0.96; $p < 0.0001$), but did not reduce CV mortality [16]. By contrast, in patients with ACS, intensive statin therapy is associated with reduced all-cause and CV mortality [18]. Niacin, fenofibrate, ezetimibe, and bile acid sequestrants may further reduce LDL cholesterol as compared to statins alone [19]. However, there is insufficient evidence that such combination therapy for LDL cholesterol lowering provides a significant increment in CV risk reduction over statin therapy alone (Table 9.1) [20, 21].

Table 9.1 Main randomized controlled trials on the management of atherogenic dyslipidemia

Trial	Population	Intervention	Effect	Outcome
FIELD ($n = 9{,}795$)	T2D with CVD	Fenofibrate or matching placebo	Fenofibrate significantly reduced TG while increasing HDL-C levels	Fenofibrate did not reduce the primary outcome of coronary events ([HR] 0.89, 95 % CI 0.75–1.05; $p = 0.16$) Only total CV events were reduced, mainly due to fewer nonfatal MI and revascularizations
ACCORD LIPID ($n = 5{,}518$)	T2D with CVD	Fenofibrate or placebo in patients who were being treated with open-label simvastatin	Fenofibrate significantly reduced TG while increasing HDL-C levels	Fenofibrate did not reduce the primary outcome of coronary events ([HR], 0.92; 95 % CI, 0.79–1.08; $p = 0.32$) No significant differences between the two study groups with respect to any secondary outcome

(continued)

Table 9.1 (continued)

Trial	Population	Intervention	Effect	Outcome
AIM-HIGH ($n=3,414$)	Established CVD	Patients randomly assigned to receive niacin or placebo	Niacin significantly increased median HDL-C and lowered TG and LDL-C	Niacin did not reduce the primary outcome of coronary events ([HR], 1.02; 95 % CI, 0.87–1.21; $p=0.79$) Similar results were observed in the subgroup of patients with DM
ILLUMINATE ($n=15,067$)	High CV risk	Torcetrapib plus atorvastatin vs. atorvastatin alone	Torcetrapib significantly increased median HDL-C while reducing LDL-C	Torcetrapib significantly increased the risk of CV events ([HR], 1.25; 95 % CI, 1.09–1.44; $p=0.001$), and death from any cause ([HR],1.58; 95 % CI, 1.14–2.19; $p=0.006$)

Table 9.1 (continued)

Trial	Population	Intervention	Effect	Outcome
Dal-OUT-COMES ($n = 15,871$)	Recent ACS	Dalcetrapib or placebo, in addition to best available evidence-based care	Dalcetrapib significantly increased median HDL-C, with minimal effect on LDL-C	As compared with placebo, dalcetrapib did not alter the risk of the primary end point ([HR], 1.04; 95 % CI, 0.93–1.16; $p = 0.52$) and did not have a significant effect on any component of the primary end point or total mortality

T2D type 2 diabetes, *CVD* cardiovascular disease, *TG* triglycerides, *HDL-C* high density lipoprotein cholesterol, *LDL-C* low density lipoprotein cholesterol, *HR* hazard ratio, *MI* myocardial infarction, *ACS* acute coronary syndrome

9.3   TGL, HDL, and Residual Vascular Risk

Albeit statins are associated with a substantial reduction of LDL cholesterol levels, CV morbidity and mortality remains high in DM patients, suggesting that other lipid components, namely TG and HDL cholesterol, may contribute to vascular risk in this setting [9]. Analyses of the HPS and CARE trials have revealed that low HDL-C levels are independently associated with CV events in patients with DM [9]. Although the TG/HDL ratio is a powerful predictor of CV outcome [22], it remains unclear whether pharmacological modulation of these lipid fractions may effectively reduce CV morbidity and mortality [2, 9]. The initial enthusiasm toward this approach came from the VA-HIT trial (*Veterans Affairs High-Density Lipoprotein Cholesterol Intervention Trial*), where chronic treatment with fenofibrate determined a 24 % reduction of CV mortality, myocardial infarction and stroke in DM patients with normal LDL levels and increased TG/HDL ratio [23]. These positive results were not confirmed in later trials. In the FIELD study (*Fenofibrate Intervention and Event Lowering in Diabetes*) treatment with fenofibrate did not reduce coronary events in 9,795 patients with T2D [24]. Fenofibrate was only associated with a modest but significant reduction of the amputation rate. The recent ACCORD lipid trial tested whether the combination fenofibrate/ simvastatin could exert further cardiovascular protection in 5,518 patients with T2D [25]. Unfortunately, this study was unable to show any reduction of the composite endpoint including fatal and nonfatal myocardial infarction, stroke, and mortality. Some authors have postulated that benefits of fibrates may be seen in patients with a marked elevation of TG/HDL ratio, but clinical data remain scarce [20]. Besides, treatment with niacin in the AIM-HIGH trial (*Atherothrombosis Intervention in Metabolic Syndrome with Low HDL/High Triglycerides*) was effective in modulating TG and HDL levels but not in reducing CV events and mortality [26]. Along the same line, treatment with the CETP inhibitors torcetrapib and dalcetrapid did not improve CV outcome despite a consistent increase of HDL levels (Table 9.1) [27].

9.4   Therapeutic Targets

Taken together, these studies do not encourage strategies aimed at modulating TG/HDL ratio. Hypertriglyceridemia should be treated with dietary and lifestyle changes [20]. Severe hypertriglyceridemia (>1,000 mg/dL) may require immediate pharmacological therapy (fibric acid derivative, niacin, or fish oil) to reduce the risk of acute pancreatitis. In the absence of severe

Table 9.2 Recommended lipid targets in patients with T2D according to cardiovascular risk

	Patients with T2D	
	Low-moderate CV risk (T2D without CVD or other major CV risk factors)	High CV risk (T2D + 1 or more major CV risk factors or CVD)
LDL-C	100 mg/dL (or 30 reduction from baseline)	≤70 mg/dL (or 40 % reduction from baseline)
Non-HDL-C	≤130 mg/dL	≤100 mg/dL
ApoB	≤90 mg/dL	≤80 mg/dL

LDL-C low density lipoprotein cholesterol, *HDL-C* high density lipoprotein cholesterol, *ApoB* apolipoprotein B

hypertriglyceridemia, therapy targeting HDL cholesterol or triglycerides lacks the strong evidence base of statin therapy. Fibrates or niacin might be used in patients intolerant to statins with marked increases in TG/HDL ratio. LDL-C remains the primary target of therapy in diabetic patients [28, 29]. However, it remains difficult to define specific cut-offs and it would be more appropriate to achieve consistent LDL reductions from baseline values. Indeed, the majority of statin trials tested specific doses of statins against placebo or other statins, rather than aiming for specific LDL cholesterol goals. RCTs generally achieved LDL cholesterol reductions of 30–40 % from baseline. Hence, LDL cholesterol lowering of this magnitude is an acceptable outcome for patients who cannot reach LDL cholesterol goals due to severe baseline elevations in LDL cholesterol and/or intolerance of maximal, or any, statin doses [20]. The use of specific LDL cut-offs in primary and secondary CVD prevention might be useful; however in many cases it is very hard to achieve the recommended targets and it more appropriate to obtain significant variations of LDL values (Table 9.2). ATP III recommendations have proposed the use of non-high-density lipoprotein cholesterol (non-HDL-C) as a secondary therapeutic target in patients with triglycerides (TG) levels >200 mg/dL. More recently non-HDL-C ≤100 mg/dL and apoB ≤80 mg/dL have been proposed as targets of therapy in high-risk patients, including those with CAD or DM plus one or more CV risk factors [30–32]. Indeed, LDL-C has shown to lose part of its predictive value in hypertriglyceridemia as a result of the increase in VLDL-C, apoB, and sd-LDL-C. Conversely, when TG levels are ≤150 mg/dL, VLDL-C represents only a small percentage of the lipoproteins pool and their concentration in the blood rarely exceeds 30 mg/dL [1].

References

1. Bosomworth NJ (2013) Approach to identifying and managing atherogenic dyslipidemia: a metabolic consequence of obesity and diabetes. Can Fam Physician 59:1169–1180
2. Arca M, Pigna G, Favoccia C (2012) Mechanisms of diabetic dyslipidemia: relevance for atherogenesis. Curr Vasc Pharmacol 10:684–686
3. Morales-Villegas E (2014) Dyslipidemia, hypertension and diabetes metaflammation. A unique mechanism for 3 risk factors. Curr Hypertens Rev. doi:10.2174/1573402110666140702091315
4. Kotseva K, Stagmo M, De Bacquer D, De Backer G, Wood D, Euroaspire II Study Group (2008) Treatment potential for cholesterol management in patients with coronary heart disease in 15 European countries: findings from the EUROASPIRE II survey. Atherosclerosis 197:710–717
5. Kotseva K, Wood D, De Backer G, De Bacquer D, Pyorala K, Keil U et al (2009) EUROASPIRE III: a survey on the lifestyle, risk factors and use of cardioprotective drug therapies in coronary patients from 22 European countries. Eur J Cardiovasc Prev Rehabil 16:121–137
6. Ginsberg HN, Tuck C (2001) Diabetes and dyslipidemia. Curr Diab Rep 1:93–95
7. Taskinen MR, Boren J (2015) New insights into the pathophysiology of dyslipidemia in type 2 diabetes. Atherosclerosis 239:483–495
8. Chapman MJ, Guerin M, Bruckert E (1998) Atherogenic, dense low-density lipoproteins. Pathophysiology and new therapeutic approaches. Eur Heart J 19(Suppl A):A24–A30

9. Hamilton SJ, Watts GF (2013) Atherogenic dyslipidemia and combination pharmacotherapy in diabetes: recent clinical trials. Rev Diabet Stud 10:191–203

10. Bays HE (2014) Lowering low-density lipoprotein cholesterol levels in patients with type 2 diabetes mellitus. Int J Gen Med 7:355–364

11. Vijayaraghavan K (2010) Treatment of dyslipidemia in patients with type 2 diabetes. Lipids Health Dis 9:144

12. Haffner SM, Alexander CM, Cook TJ, Boccuzzi SJ, Musliner TA, Pedersen TR et al (1999) Reduced coronary events in simvastatin-treated patients with coronary heart disease and diabetes or impaired fasting glucose levels: subgroup analyses in the Scandinavian Simvastatin Survival Study. Arch Intern Med 159:2661–2667

13. Goldberg RB, Mellies MJ, Sacks FM, Moye LA, Howard BV, Howard WJ et al (1998) Cardiovascular events and their reduction with pravastatin in diabetic and glucose-intolerant myocardial infarction survivors with average cholesterol levels: subgroup analyses in the cholesterol and recurrent events (CARE) trial. The Care Investigators. Circulation 98:2513–2519

14. Sever PS, Dahlof B, Poulter NR, Wedel H, Beevers G, Caulfield M et al (2003) Prevention of coronary and stroke events with atorvastatin in hypertensive patients who have average or lower-than-average cholesterol concentrations, in the Anglo-Scandinavian Cardiac Outcomes Trial–Lipid Lowering Arm (ASCOT-LLA): a multicentre randomised controlled trial. Lancet 361:1149–1158

15. Colhoun HM, Betteridge DJ, Durrington PN, Hitman GA, Neil HA, Livingstone SJ et al (2004) Primary prevention of cardiovascular disease with atorvastatin in type 2 diabetes in the Collaborative Atorvastatin Diabetes Study (CARDS): multicentre randomised placebo-controlled trial. Lancet 364:685–696

16. Kearney PM, Blackwell L, Collins R, Keech A, Simes J, Peto R et al (2008) Efficacy of cholesterol-lowering therapy in 18,686 people with diabetes in 14 randomised trials of statins: a meta-analysis. Lancet 371:117–125

17. Shepherd J, Barter P, Carmena R, Deedwania P, Fruchart JC, Haffner S et al (2006) Effect of lowering LDL cholesterol substantially below currently recommended levels in patients with coronary heart disease and diabetes: the Treating to New Targets (TNT) study. Diabetes Care 29:1220–1226

18. Cannon CP, Steinberg BA, Murphy SA, Mega JL, Braunwald E (2006) Meta-analysis of cardiovascular outcomes trials comparing intensive versus moderate statin therapy. J Am Coll Cardiol 48:438–445

19. Kumar A, Singh V (2010) Atherogenic dyslipidemia and diabetes mellitus: what's new in the management arena? Vasc Health Risk Manag 6:665–669
20. American Diabetes Association (2014) Standards of medical care in diabetes – 2014. Diabetes Care 37(Suppl 1):S14–S80
21. Ryden L, Grant PJ, Anker SD, Berne C, Cosentino F, Danchin N et al (2013) ESC Guidelines on diabetes, pre-diabetes, and cardiovascular diseases developed in collaboration with the EASD: the Task Force on diabetes, pre-diabetes, and cardiovascular diseases of the European Society of Cardiology (ESC) and developed in collaboration with the European Association for the Study of Diabetes (EASD). Eur Heart J 34:3035–3087
22. Arca M, Montali A, Valiante S, Campagna F, Pigna G, Paoletti V et al (2007) Usefulness of atherogenic dyslipidemia for predicting cardiovascular risk in patients with angiographically defined coronary artery disease. Am J Cardiol 100:1511–1516
23. Rubins HB, Robins SJ, Collins D, Fye CL, Anderson JW, Elam MB et al (1999) Gemfibrozil for the secondary prevention of coronary heart disease in men with low levels of high-density lipoprotein cholesterol. Veterans Affairs High-Density Lipoprotein Cholesterol Intervention Trial Study Group. N Engl J Med 341:410–418
24. Keech A, Simes RJ, Barter P, Best J, Scott R, Taskinen MR et al (2005) Effects of long-term fenofibrate therapy on cardiovascular events in 9795 people with type 2 diabetes mellitus (the FIELD study): randomised controlled trial. Lancet 366:1849–1861
25. Ginsberg HN, Elam MB, Lovato LC, Crouse JR 3rd, Leiter LA, Linz P et al (2010) Effects of combination lipid therapy in type 2 diabetes mellitus. N Engl J Med 362:1563–1574
26. Boden WE, Probstfield JL, Anderson T, Chaitman BR, Desvignes-Nickens P, Koprowicz K et al (2011) Niacin in patients with low HDL cholesterol levels receiving intensive statin therapy. N Engl J Med 365:2255–2267
27. Landmesser U, von Eckardstein A, Kastelein J, Deanfield J, Luscher TF (2012) Increasing high-density lipoprotein cholesterol by cholesteryl ester transfer protein-inhibition: a rocky road and lessons learned? The early demise of the dal-HEART programme. Eur Heart J 33:1712–1715
28. Ali YS, Linton MF, Fazio S (2008) Targeting cardiovascular risk in patients with diabetes: management of dyslipidemia. Curr Opin Endocrinol Diabetes Obes 15:142–146
29. Tripolt NJ, Sourij H (2014) New American College of Cardiology and American Heart Association cholesterol treatment guidelines: subjects with type 2 diabetes are under treated with high-intensity statins. Diabet Med 31:879–880

30. de Nijs T, Sniderman A, de Graaf J (2013) ApoB versus non-HDL-cholesterol: diagnosis and cardiovascular risk management. Crit Rev Clin Lab Sci 50:163–171
31. Ray KK, Kastelein JJ, Boekholdt SM, Nicholls SJ, Khaw KT, Ballantyne CM et al (2014) The ACC/AHA 2013 guideline on the treatment of blood cholesterol to reduce atherosclerotic cardiovascular disease risk in adults: the good the bad and the uncertain: a comparison with ESC/EAS guidelines for the management of dyslipidaemias 2011. Eur Heart J 35:960–968
32. Brunzell JD, Davidson M, Furberg CD, Goldberg RB, Howard BV, Stein JH et al (2008) Lipoprotein management in patients with cardio-metabolic risk: consensus conference report from the American Diabetes Association and the American College of Cardiology Foundation. J Am Coll Cardiol 51:1512–1524

Chapter 10
Arterial Hypertension

10.1 Prevalence and Pathophysiology

Arterial hypertension (AH) is a common finding in patients with type 2 diabetes (T2D) [1]. DM people have indeed a three- to sixfold higher risk to develop AH as compared to non-DM subjects [2]. Moreover, in DM patients, masked hypertension is not infrequent and monitoring 24-h ambulatory BP may be a useful approach. In T1D, AH is mainly the result of nephropathy whereas in T2D patients abdominal obesity, reduced physical activity, hyperinsulinemia, sympathetic tone as well as activation of the renin-angiotensin-aldosterone (RAAS) system are the main mechanisms involved [3–5]. Different factors clustering in diabetic patients (i.e., renal dysfunction, dyslipidemia, obesity) significantly contribute to raise blood pressure (BP) values. This aspect explains why an intensive therapeutic regimen including a combination of two to three antihypertensive agents is often required to treat AH in diabetic patients [6].

F. Paneni, F. Cosentino, *Diabetes and Cardiovascular Disease:* 115
A Guide to Clinical Management, DOI 10.1007/978-3-319-17762-5_10,
© Springer International Publishing Switzerland 2015

10.2   Clinical Evidence

The ABCD study (*Appropriate Blood pressure Control in Diabetes*) has shown that achieving BP target determines a significant reduction of cardiovascular (CV) events over a 4-year follow-up (Table 10.1) [7]. In a subgroup of 1,148 hypertensive patients with T2D, the UKPDS investigators aimed to estimate the benefits of tight versus less-tight BP control, to ascertain the impact of BP lowering and to compare the beneficial effects of an angiotensin converting enzyme (ACE) inhibitor (captopril) versus a β-blocker (atenolol). After a median follow-up of 8.4 years, tight BP control was associated with a significant decrease of BP values as compared to conventional therapy (144/82 mmHg vs. 154/87 mmHg). Such an approach resulted in 44 % and 32 % reduction of stroke and DM-related death, respectively. However, the 10-year post-monitoring follow-up of this substudy demonstrated that intensive BP lowering was not associated with a sustained and significant reduction in CV outcomes [8]. The investigators concluded that antihypertensive treatment is of key importance in hypertensive patients with DM, but their benefits are not sustained over time. The ACCORD study has shown that intensive BP lowering (119 vs. 134 mmHg) for 5 years did not reduce CV events while increasing side effects such as hypotension and renal dysfunction (3.3 vs. 1.3 %), as assessed by glomerular filtration rate (GFR) [9]. A recent meta-analysis including 13 randomized trials with more than 37,000 patients has shown that a BP reduction < 130 mmHg is associated with a 20 % increase in the risk of adverse CV events, indicating that lowering BP is beneficial within certain BP ranges but should be performed with caution, especially in patients with DM [10].

Table 10.1 Randomized controlled trials on blood pressure reduction and cardiovascular risk in patients with diabetes

Study/No. of pts	Duration (years)	BP control		Therapy	Outcome	RR (%)
		Less tight	Tight			
SHEP/583	5	155/72*	143/68*	Chlorthalidone	Stroke	NS
					CV events	34
					Coronary disease	56
Syst-Eur/492	2	162/82	153/78	Nifedipine	Stroke	69
					CV events	62
HOT/1,501	3	144/85*	140/81*	Felodipine	CV events	51
					MI	50
					Stroke	NS
					CV death	67
UKPDS/1,148	8.4	154/87	144/82	Captopril or atenolol	Diabetes-related endpoints	34
					Death	37
					Stroke	44
					Microvascular endpoint	37

(continued)

Table 10.1 (continued)

Study/No. of pts	Duration (years)	BP control		Therapy	Outcome	RR (%)
		Less tight	Tight			
HOPE, Micro-HOPE/ 3,577	4.5	SBP reduction (2.4 mmHg), DBP reduction (1.0 mmHg)	–	Ramipril vs. placebo	CV events	25
					CV death	37
					MI	22
					Stroke	33
					All-cause death	24
					New-onset diabetes	34
CAPP/572	7	155/89 vs. 153/88	–	Captopril vs. diuretics or BB	Fatal and nonfatal MI+ stroke + CV death	41
IDNT/1,715	2.6	≤135/85	–	Irbesartan vs. amlodipine or placebo	Renal failure+all-cause death	23 (vs. amlodipine) 20 (vs. placebo)
IRMA/590	2	144/83143/ 83141/83	–	Irbesartan 150 mg or 300 mg vs. placebo	Diabetic nephropathy	35 (150 mg) 65 (300 mg)

Study/N	Follow-up	BP		Comparison	Endpoint	Result
RENAAL/ 1,513	3.4	152/82 vs. 153/82	—	Losartan vs. placebo	Renal dysfunction	25
					End-stage renal disease	28
LIFE/1,195	4.8	146/79 vs. 148/79	—	Losartan vs. atenolol	Death	NS
					CV events	22
					Total death in diabetics	39
					New-onset diabetes	25
INSIGHT/ 6,321	4	145/82 vs. 144/82		Nifedipine 30 mg or idrocloroti-azide 25 mg + amiloride 2.5 mg	CV death+	NS
					MI+HF+stroke	
					Composite primary endpoint including all-cause mortality	24 (nifedipine)
VALUE/ 15,245	4	139/79 vs. 137/78	—	Valsartan vs. amlodipine	Cardiac morbidity and mortality	NS
ASCOT-BPLA/ 19,237 (13 % diabetics)	5.5	130/80 in 32 % of patients in both groups	—	Amlodipine ± per-indopril vs. atenolol ± thi-azide diuretic	Fatal and nonfatal MI	NS

(continued)

Table 10.1 (continued)

Study/No. of pts	Duration (years)	BP control		Therapy	Outcome	RR (%)
		Less tight	Tight			
UKPDS/884	10 (partial monitoring)	No differences	–		Diabetes-related endpoints	NS
					Death	NS
					Stroke	NS
					Microvascular endpoints	NS
ADVANCE/ 11,140	4.3	136/73 vs. 140/73	–	Perindopril+ indapamide vs. placebo	Total mortality	14
					Total coronary events	14
					Major vascular events	9
					New-onset microalbuminuria	21
ONTARGET/ 25,620	4.8	Variation of 0.9/0.6 mmHg e 2.4/1.4 mmHg in telmisartan and combination therapy	–	Ramipril vs. telmisartan vs. combination	Composite endpoint of CV death, MI, stroke, or HF hospitalization	NS

Trial/N		Variation		Comparison	Endpoint	Result
TRANSCEND/ 5,926 (35 % diabetics)	4.8	Variation of 3.2/1.8 mmHg	–	Telmisartan vs. placebo	Composite endpoint of CV death, MI, stroke, or HF hospitalization	NS
ACCORD/ 4,733	4.7	119.3 vs. 133.5 mmHg	–	Intensive vs. conventional therapy	Composite endpoint of CV death, MI, stroke, or HF hospitalization	NS
ROADMAP/ 4,447	3.2	Variation of 3.1/1.9 mmHg	–	Olmesartan vs. placebo	CV events Total death in diabetics New-onset diabetes	NS 34 56
ALTITUDE/ 8,561	3.9	Variation of 1.3/0.6 mmHg	–	ACEs vs. aliskiren + ACEs	Composite endpoint of fatal/nonfatal CV events, HF, ESRD	NS

*$p < 0.05$

CV cardiovascular, *NS* not significant, *MI* myocardial infarction, *ESRD* end-stage renal disease, *BP* blood pressure

10.3   Blood Pressure Targets in People with Diabetes

At present, there is no clear evidence of benefits from initiating antihypertensive treatment at SBP levels <140 mmHg (high normal BP) nor there is evidence of benefits from aiming at targets <130 mmHg [11]. Intensive BP control did not improve diabetic retinopathy in normotensive and hypertensive patients in the *Action in Diabetes and Vascular Disease: Preterax and Diamicron-MR Controlled Evaluation* (ADVANCE) trial, and in the normotensive type-1 diabetics of the *DIabetic REtinopathy Candesartan Trials* (DIRECT) [12, 13]. Moreover, antihypertensive drugs do not appear to substantially affect neuropathy [11]. Taken together, studies available so far suggest that people with DM and hypertension should be treated to a systolic blood pressure (SBP) goal of <140 mmHg and a DBP<85 mmHg (Table 10.2) [11]. Lower systolic targets, such as <130 mmHg, may be appropriate for certain individuals, namely younger patients [14]. Lifestyle measures should be undertaken in all DM patients with BP values >120/80 mmHg. Patients with confirmed BP higher than 140/80 mmHg should, in addition to lifestyle therapy, have prompt initiation and timely subsequent titration of pharmacological therapy to achieve BP goals [14].

10.4   Antihypertensive Drugs

The choice of antihypertensive drugs should be based on efficacy and tolerability. All the available BP lowering drugs are effective but their use vary according to patient characteristics including age, heart rate, renal function, presence of coronary artery disease, and obesity [11, 15].

Table 10.2 Blood pressure targets in diabetic people according to age and the presence of renal or cardiovascular disease

	Young <40 years	Elderly >75 years	Renal dysfunction (GFR <60 ml/min) or albuminuria (>300 mg/24 h)	Coronary disease/heart failure
Systolic blood pressure (mmHg)	<130	<150	<140	<140
Diastolic blood pressure (mmHg)	<80	<85	<85	<85
Antihypertensive agent of choice	ACEs/ARBs/DRI	Diuretics, CCB, BB	ACEi/ARB/DRI	ACEi/ARBs/DRI, BB, diuretics
Comments	Perform BP monitoring	Ideal SBP target 150–140 mmHg	Monitor serum creatinine; avoid combination therapy with RAAS blockers	Ideal SBP target 140–130 mmHg

ACEs angiotensin converting enzyme inhibitors, *ARBs* angiotensin receptor blockers, *DRI* direct renin inhibitors, *CCB* calcium channel blockers, *BB* beta blockers

10.4.1 RAAS Inhibitors

RAAS is activated by hyperglycemia in DM patients, and its antagonism is associated with a consistent reduction in micro- and macrovascular complications [5, 16]. Beyond their BP lowering effect, RAAS inhibiting drugs antagonize vascular inflammation and remodeling, with a subsequent reduction of reparative fibrosis and vascular stiffness [17, 18]. Such changes are sustained and strongly contribute to a reduction in peripheral resistance and BP. Hence, pleiotropic effects of RAAS inhibitors that go beyond BP reduction may provide the rationale for a legacy effect of such an antihypertensive strategy in DM. Pharmacological suppression of RAAS prevents left ventricular hypertrophy, reduces left atrial volume and risk of atrial fibrillation in DM patients [19]. Moreover, this class of drugs is highly effective in preventing microalbuminuria and renal dysfunction [16]. In the HOPE study, treatment with ramipril significantly reduced the combined endpoint of myocardial infarction, stroke, and CV death [20]. Similarly, the ARB losartan reduced CV mortality as compared with the beta blocker atenolol in the DM patients of the LIFE study [21]. Routine administration of a fixed combination of perindopril and indapamide to more than 11,000 patients with T2D significantly reduced macrovascular events and CV mortality by 9 % and 18 %, respectively [22]. DM patients receiving fosinopril had a significantly lower risk of acute MI, stroke, or hospitalized angina than those receiving amlodipine in the FACET trial [23]. Similarly, in the ABCD study, enalapril significantly improved CV outcomes in DM patients, and was associated with fewer MIs than treatment with nisoldipine (adjusted HR = 7 for nisoldipine vs. enalapril; 95 % CI, 2.3–21.4) [7].

10.4.2 RAAS and Renal Outcomes in Type 2 Diabetes

RAAS inhibitors have been shown to be more effective in reducing albuminuria than other classes of antihypertensive drugs, as a consequence of angiotensin II blockade. The use of irbesartan almost abolished renal microvascular complications compared with conventional antihypertensive therapy in patients with T2D [24]. Valsartan and losartan reduced renal complications in a BP-independent manner in the MARVAL and RENAAL trials [25, 26]. Similarly, the micro-HOPE trial demonstrated that the use of ramipril significantly decreased the incidence of diabetic nephropathy [27]. Also in the BENEDICT study, ACE inhibitors limited the development of microalbuminuria in a relatively small cohort of patients [28]. More recently, the use of olmesartan resulted in a 23 % reduction in the occurrence of microalbuminuria in the ROADMAP trial, and BP targets were achieved by more than 80 % of the 5,000 DM patients enrolled [29]. However, olmesartan did not improve CV morbidity and mortality in this trial. More recently, the direct renin inhibitor aliskiren in combination with losartan significantly reduced proteinuria as compared to monotherapy (20 % vs. 12.5 %, $p<0.001$) [30]. By contrast, the association of aliskiren with losartan is associated with increased CV and renal events in high-risk DM patients [31].

10.4.3 ACEs/ARBs Treatment and New-Onset Diabetes

Another important effect of RAAS blockers is that these drugs may reduce the incidence of diabetes. The recently published

Nateglinide and Valsartan Impaired Glucose Tolerance Outcomes Research (NAVIGATOR) trial showed that the use of valsartan along with lifestyle modifications for 5 years led to a relative reduction of 14 % in the incidence of DM in patients with impaired glucose tolerance and CVD or risk factors [32]. Elliott and colleagues showed that ARBs and ACE inhibitors were more effective in preventing the incidence of new DM than diuretics, calcium antagonists, and β-blockers [33]. More recently, a large and updated meta-analysis showed that ARBs prevent new-onset DM as compared to other active antihypertensive treatments [34]. Taken together with several other reports, all these findings strongly support the advantage of RAAS blockade as compared with conventional antihypertensive drugs in diabetics [11].

10.4.4   Calcium Channel Blockers, Beta Blockers, Diuretics

Calcium channel blockers are also effective to reach BP target in DM patients. In Syst-Eur and HOT studies, high-dose CCBs in T2D patients have strongly reduced the rate of ischemic stroke and CV mortality [35, 36]. Diuretics are powerful BP lowering agents, particularly in the elderly. The SHEP trial has shown that the use of a thiazide diuretic was very effective to achieve BP goals and reduce CV mortality [37]. Finally, beta blockers though potentially impairing insulin sensitivity are useful for BP control in combination therapy, particularly in patients with coronary heart disease and heart failure [11]. Current guidelines have recently outlined that pharmacological therapy for patients with DM and hypertension should comprise a regimen that includes either an ACE inhibitor or an ARB. Multiple-drug therapy (two or more agents at maximal doses) is generally required to achieve BP targets. If ACE inhibitors, ARBs, or diuretics are used, serum creatinine, GFR as well as serum potassium levels should be monitored [11].

10.5   Resistant Hypertension and Renal Sympathetic Denervation

Renal sympathetic denervation (RSDN) may represent a promising therapeutic approach to treat AH in patients with DM [38]. This is a minimally invasive, endovascular catheter based procedure using radiofrequency ablation or ultrasound ablation aimed at treating resistant hypertension. The latter represents a common clinical problem in patients with obesity and T2D, with a prevalence ranging from 20 to 30 %. The prognosis of resistant hypertension is unknown, but CV risk is undoubtedly increased as patients often have a history of long-standing, severe hypertension complicated by multiple other CV risk factors such as obesity, sleep apnea, and chronic kidney disease. During renal denervation nerves in the wall of the renal artery are ablated by applying radiofrequency pulses or ultrasound to the renal arteries. This causes reduction of sympathetic afferent and efferent activity to the kidney and subsequent BP reduction. Early data from randomized clinical trials without sham controls were promising and demonstrated large BP reductions in patients with treatment-resistant hypertension [39]. A pilot study on 50 hypertensive patients demonstrated that renal denervation improves glucose metabolism and insulin sensitivity in addition to a significant effect on BP. This novel procedure may therefore provide protection in patients with resistant hypertension and metabolic disorders at high cardiovascular risk [40]. However, in 2014 the SYMPLICITY HTN-3 study, a prospective, single-blind, randomized, sham-controlled clinical trial failed to confirm a beneficial effect on BP [41]. Further studies are needed to confirm the effectiveness of this strategy.

References

1. Grossman Y, Shlomai G, Grossman E (2014) Treating hypertension in type 2 diabetes. Expert Opin Pharmacother 15:2131–2140
2. Vijan S (2014) Diabetes: treating hypertension. BMJ Clin Evid 06:608
3. Lastra G, Syed S, Kurukulasuriya LR, Manrique C, Sowers JR (2014) Type 2 diabetes mellitus and hypertension: an update. Endocrinol Metab Clin North Am 43:103–122
4. Pieske B, Wachter R (2008) Impact of diabetes and hypertension on the heart. Curr Opin Cardiol 23:340–349
5. Volpe M, Cosentino F, Tocci G, Palano F, Paneni F (2011) Antihypertensive therapy in diabetes: the legacy effect and RAAS blockade. Curr Hypertens Rep 13:318–324
6. Bayliss G, Weinrauch LA, D'Elia JA (2014) Resistant hypertension in diabetes mellitus. Curr Diab Rep 14:516
7. Mehler PS, Coll JR, Estacio R, Esler A, Schrier RW, Hiatt WR (2003) Intensive blood pressure control reduces the risk of cardiovascular events in patients with peripheral arterial disease and type 2 diabetes. Circulation 107:753–756
8. Holman RR, Paul SK, Bethel MA, Neil HA, Matthews DR (2008) Long-term follow-up after tight control of blood pressure in type 2 diabetes. N Engl J Med 359:1565–1576
9. Cushman WC, Evans GW, Byington RP, Goff DC Jr, Grimm RH Jr, Cutler JA et al (2010) Effects of intensive blood-pressure control in type 2 diabetes mellitus. N Engl J Med 362:1575–1585
10. Bangalore S, Kumar S, Lobach I, Messerli FH (2011) Blood pressure targets in subjects with type 2 diabetes mellitus/impaired fasting glucose: observations from traditional and bayesian random-effects meta-analyses of randomized trials. Circulation 123:2799–2810
11. Mancia G, Fagard R, Narkiewicz K, Redon J, Zanchetti A, Bohm M et al (2013) 2013 ESH/ESC guidelines for the management of arterial hypertension: the Task Force for the Management of Arterial Hypertension of the European Society of Hypertension (ESH) and of the European Society of Cardiology (ESC). Eur Heart J 34:2159–2219
12. Beulens JW, Patel A, Vingerling JR, Cruickshank JK, Hughes AD, Stanton A et al (2009) Effects of blood pressure lowering and intensive glucose control on the incidence and progression of retinopathy in patients with type 2 diabetes mellitus: a randomised controlled trial. Diabetologia 52:2027–2036
13. Chaturvedi N, Porta M, Klein R, Orchard T, Fuller J, Parving HH et al (2008) Effect of candesartan on prevention (DIRECT-Prevent 1) and

progression (DIRECT-Protect 1) of retinopathy in type 1 diabetes: randomised, placebo-controlled trials. Lancet 372:1394–1402

14. American Diabetes Association (2014) Standards of medical care in diabetes – 2014. Diabetes Care 37(Suppl 1):S14–S80

15. Ryden L, Grant PJ, Anker SD, Berne C, Cosentino F, Danchin N et al (2013) ESC Guidelines on diabetes, pre-diabetes, and cardiovascular diseases developed in collaboration with the EASD: the Task Force on diabetes, pre-diabetes, and cardiovascular diseases of the European Society of Cardiology (ESC) and developed in collaboration with the European Association for the Study of Diabetes (EASD). Eur Heart J 34:3035–3087

16. Hsueh WA, Wyne K (2011) Renin-Angiotensin-aldosterone system in diabetes and hypertension. J Clin Hypertens (Greenwich) 13: 224–237

17. Steckelings UM, Rompe F, Kaschina E, Unger T (2009) The evolving story of the RAAS in hypertension, diabetes and CV disease: moving from macrovascular to microvascular targets. Fundam Clin Pharmacol 23:693–703

18. Jandeleit-Dahm K, Cooper ME (2006) Hypertension and diabetes: role of the renin-angiotensin system. Endocrinol Metab Clin North Am 35:469–490

19. Sciarretta S, Paneni F, Palano F, Chin D, Tocci G, Rubattu S et al (2009) Role of the renin-angiotensin-aldosterone system and inflammatory processes in the development and progression of diastolic dysfunction. Clin Sci (Lond) 116:467–477

20. Heart Outcomes Prevention Evaluation Study Investigators (2000) Effects of ramipril on cardiovascular and microvascular outcomes in people with diabetes mellitus: results of the HOPE study and MICRO-HOPE substudy. Lancet 355:253–259

21. Sica DA (2002) Cardiovascular morbidity and mortality in patients with diabetes in the Losartan Intervention For Endpoint reduction in hypertension study (LIFE): a randomised trial against atenolol. Curr Hypertens Rep 4:321–323

22. Patel A, MacMahon S, Chalmers J, Neal B, Woodward M, Billot L et al (2007) Effects of a fixed combination of perindopril and indapamide on macrovascular and microvascular outcomes in patients with type 2 diabetes mellitus (the ADVANCE trial): a randomised controlled trial. Lancet 370:829–840

23. Tatti P, Pahor M, Byington RP, Di Mauro P, Guarisco R, Strollo G et al (1998) Outcome results of the Fosinopril Versus Amlodipine Cardiovascular Events Randomized Trial (FACET) in patients with hypertension and NIDDM. Diabetes Care 21:597–603

24. Parving HH, Lehnert H, Brochner-Mortensen J, Gomis R, Andersen S, Arner P et al (2001) The effect of irbesartan on the development of diabetic nephropathy in patients with type 2 diabetes. N Engl J Med 345:870–878

25. Viberti G, Wheeldon NM (2002) MicroAlbuminuria Reduction With VALsartan (MARVAL) Study Investigators. Microalbuminuria reduction with valsartan in patients with type 2 diabetes mellitus: a blood pressure-independent effect. Circulation 106:672–678

26. Brenner BM, Cooper ME, de Zeeuw D, Keane WF, Mitch WE, Parving HH et al (2001) Effects of losartan on renal and cardiovascular outcomes in patients with type 2 diabetes and nephropathy. N Engl J Med 345:861–869

27. Heinig RE (2002) What should the role of ACE inhibitors be in the treatment of diabetes? Lessons from HOPE and MICRO-HOPE. Diabetes Obes Metab 4(Suppl 1):S19–S25

28. Benedict Group (2003) The BErgamo NEphrologic DIabetes Complications Trial (BENEDICT): design and baseline characteristics. Control Clin Trials 24:442–461

29. Grassi G, Mancia G (2011) Prevention of microalbuminuria in diabetes mellitus: results of the ROADMAP trial. Curr Hypertens Rep 13: 265–267

30. Parving HH, Persson F, Lewis JB, Lewis EJ, Hollenberg NK (2008) Aliskiren combined with losartan in type 2 diabetes and nephropathy. N Engl J Med 358:2433–2446

31. Parving HH, Brenner BM, McMurray JJ, de Zeeuw D, Haffner SM, Solomon SD et al (2012) Cardiorenal end points in a trial of aliskiren for type 2 diabetes. N Engl J Med 367:2204–2213

32. McMurray JJ, Holman RR, Haffner SM, Bethel MA, Holzhauer B, Hua TA et al (2010) Effect of valsartan on the incidence of diabetes and cardiovascular events. N Engl J Med 362:1477–1490

33. Elliott WJ, Meyer PM (2007) Incident diabetes in clinical trials of antihypertensive drugs: a network meta-analysis. Lancet 369:201–207

34. Tocci G, Paneni F, Palano F, Sciarretta S, Ferrucci A, Kurtz T et al (2011) Angiotensin-converting enzyme inhibitors, angiotensin II receptor blockers and diabetes: a meta-analysis of placebo-controlled clinical trials. Am J Hypertens 24:582–590

35. McFarlane SI, Farag A, Sowers J (2003) Calcium antagonists in patients with type 2 diabetes and hypertension. Cardiovasc Drug Rev 21:105–118

36. Aksnes TA, Skarn SN, Kjeldsen SE (2012) Treatment of hypertension in diabetes: what is the best therapeutic option? Expert Rev Cardiovasc Ther 10:727–734

37. Curb JD, Pressel SL, Cutler JA, Savage PJ, Applegate WB, Black H et al (1996) Effect of diuretic-based antihypertensive treatment on cardiovascular disease risk in older diabetic patients with isolated systolic hypertension. Systolic Hypertension in the Elderly Program Cooperative Research Group. JAMA 276:1886–1892
38. Mahfoud F, Ewen S, Ukena C, Linz D, Sobotka PA, Cremers B et al (2013) Expanding the indication spectrum: renal denervation in diabetes. EuroIntervention 9(Suppl R):R117–R121
39. Esler MD, Krum H, Sobotka PA, Schlaich MP, Schmieder RE, Bohm M et al (2010) Renal sympathetic denervation in patients with treatment-resistant hypertension (The Symplicity HTN-2 Trial): a randomised controlled trial. Lancet 376:1903–1909
40. Mahfoud F, Schlaich M, Kindermann I, Ukena C, Cremers B, Brandt MC et al (2011) Effect of renal sympathetic denervation on glucose metabolism in patients with resistant hypertension: a pilot study. Circulation 123:1940–1946
41. Bhatt DL, Kandzari DE, O'Neill WW, D'Agostino R, Flack JM, Katzen BT et al (2014) A controlled trial of renal denervation for resistant hypertension. N Engl J Med 370:1393–1401

Chapter 11
Antiplatelet Therapy

11.1 Enhanced Platelet Reactivity in Diabetes

High platelet reactivity strongly contributes to recurrent coronary events and mortality in patients with diabetes (DM) [1]. Insulin resistance in T2D patients favors calcium accumulation upon basal conditions by suppressing the IRS-1/Akt pathway [2]. This latter mechanism contributes to explain why platelets from DM patients show faster response and increased aggregation compared with those from healthy subjects [3]. Increased Ca^{2+} content, thrombin stimulation as well as interaction with von Willebrand factor (vWF) via GpIIb/IIIa receptor lead to platelet shape change, granule release, and aggregation [4]. Moreover, platelet reactivity and excretion of thromboxane metabolites are increased in obese patients with insulin resistance, and this phenomenon is reversed by weight loss or 3-week treatment with pioglitazone [5]. Body weight as well as impaired insulin sensitivity may also account for the faster recovery of cyclooxygenase activity despite aspirin treatment. Indeed, higher body mass index was an independent predictor of inadequate suppression of thromboxane biosynthesis in non-DM subjects treated with aspirin [6].

F. Paneni, F. Cosentino, *Diabetes and Cardiovascular Disease:*
A Guide to Clinical Management, DOI 10.1007/978-3-319-17762-5_11,
© Springer International Publishing Switzerland 2015

11.2   Aspirin

Aspirin hampers platelet activation and aggregation by suppressing the biosynthesis of thromboxane A_2 through irreversible inactivation of cyclooxygenase 1 (COX-1). Although platelet reactivity is a major feature of DM patients, the benefits of aspirin in T2D subjects without established atherosclerotic vascular disease remain inconclusive. At present, current recommendations by the US Preventive Service and the American College of Chest Physician suggest the use of low-dose aspirin (75–162 mg once daily) for primary prevention of CVD [7, 8]. This notion is mainly based on a comprehensive meta-analysis of primary prevention trials showing a small benefit of aspirin reduction of nonfatal myocardial infarction (about 5 events per 10,000 patients) offset by a similar increase in gastrointestinal hemorrhage (3 events per 10,000 patients) [9]. Evidence collected so far in the DM population does not seem to be compelling. The *Japanese Primary Prevention of Atherosclerosis with Aspirin for Diabetes* (JAPAD) Trial included 2,539 patients with DM and no history of atherosclerotic disease [10]. There was a nonsignificant 20 % reduction in atherosclerotic events (fatal and nonfatal MI, fatal and nonfatal stroke, and peripheral artery disease). Similarly, in the *Prevention of Progression of Arterial Disease and Diabetes* (POPADAD) trial, 1,276 adults with T2D and an ankle-brachial index of <1.0 were randomized to daily aspirin or placebo [11]. In this study, there was no significant difference in the composite outcome of death from CHD or stroke, nonfatal MI or stroke, or above-ankle amputation for critical limb ischemia; or any of its individual components. An updated meta-analysis of aspirin including three trials conducted specifically in patients with DM, and six other trials in which DM patients represent a subgroup, demonstrated a trend toward a 9 % reduction in CVD events (RR 0.91; 95 % CI 0.79–1.05, Fig. 11.1) [12]. On the other hand, aspirin treatment is associated with a 55 % increase in bleeding risk, mainly gastrointestinal, as shown by a meta-analysis of primary prevention trials

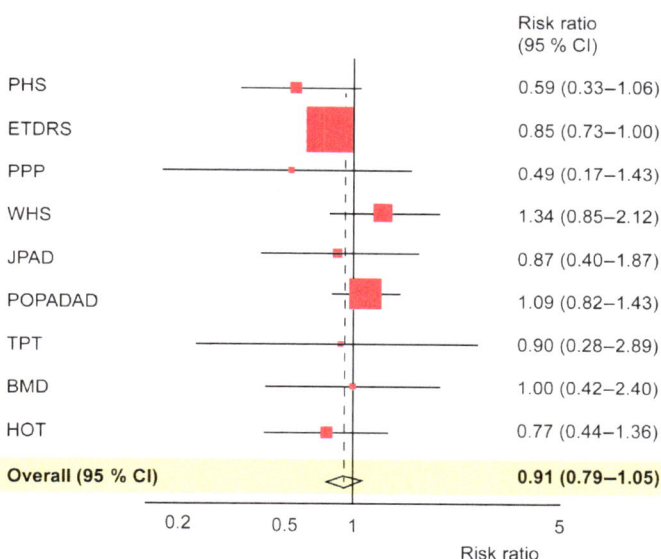

Fig. 11.1 Meta-analysis of trials examining the effects of aspirin on coronary heart events in patients with diabetes (Modified from Pignone et al. [12])

conducted in patients with and without DM [9]. Aspirin-related hemorrhagic risk is likely underestimated since patients at high risk of gastrointestinal bleeding were excluded in major clinical trials. Based on the limited data and small, if any, benefit, the use of low-dose aspirin is suggested for DM patients at increased cardiovascular risk (10-year risk >10 %), based on DM-based risk calculators such as the UKPDS Risk Engine [13, 14]. This includes mostly men aged >50 years or women aged >60 years who have at least one additional major risk factor (family history of CVD, hypertension, smoking, dyslipidemia, or albuminuria). Considering the balance between the potential benefit and hazard of aspirin in primary prevention, aspirin should not be recommended for CVD prevention for adults with DM at low CVD risk (such as in men aged <50 years and women aged <60 years with no major additional CVD risk factors), since the potential adverse effects from bleeding likely offset the potential benefits [15]. Ongoing primary prevention trials in DM patients (ASCEND and ACCEPT-D) will help to define the risk/benefit of low-dose aspirin in primary prevention of CVD [16, 17]. Taken together, evidence available so far suggest that DM per se may not be enough to warrant low-dose aspirin therapy, but use of aspirin may be acceptable when the CV risk surmounts the 1 % per year [18]. In secondary prevention, aspirin treatment is similarly effective in patients with and without DM. Data from the Antiplatelet Trialists' Collaboration on more than 45,000 DM patients showed that antiplatelet therapy reduces major vascular events by 25 % [9]. Hence, the use of aspirin at a dose of 75–160 mg is highly recommended in DM patients with a history of CVD [15].

11.3   Clopidogrel

ADP plays an important role in the genesis of physiological platelet-rich hemostatic plugs as well as in the formation of pathological arterial thrombi [2]. ADP released from platelet dense-granules as well as injured cells binds to two platelet G-protein-coupled receptors, the $P2Y_1$ and $P2Y_{12}$ receptors, thus triggering platelet aggregation. $P2Y_{12}$ plays a central role in amplification and stabilization of ADP-induced platelet aggregation. It is also involved in platelet secretion induced by strong agonists. Blockade of this receptor represents a valid therapeutic strategy to prevent atherothrombotic complications in DM patients [15]. Clopidogrel is an irreversible inhibitor of $P2Y_{12}$ with proved clinical efficacy in ACS, stroke as well as during chronic follow-up [19]. In the *Clopidogrel versus Aspirin in Patients at Risk of Ischemic Events* (CAPRIE) trial, 19,185 patients with CAD, cerebrovascular disease, or peripheral artery disease were randomized to aspirin or clopidogrel [20]. A modest 0.5 % absolute annual risk reduction was noted. In the diabetic subgroup of 1,952 patients, the absolute risk reduction was 2.1 %, significantly larger than in subjects without DM [21]. However, in The *Clopidogrel for High Atherothrombotic Risk and Ischemic Stabilization, Management, and Avoidance* (CHARISMA) trial of patients with established atherosclerosis or multiple risk factors for atherosclerosis, the addition of clopidogrel to aspirin was no more effective than aspirin alone in prevention of the composite endpoint of CV death, MI, and stroke [22]. The *Clopidogrel in Unstable Angina to Prevent Recurrent Events* (CURE) trial demonstrated benefit in reducing the composite of CV death, nonfatal MI, and stroke with the addition of clopidogrel to aspirin in both non-DM and DM patients with ACS [23].

11.4   Prasugrel

Prasugrel is a third-generation thienopyridine recently approved for clinical use in ACS patients undergoing PCI. It is orally administered and, like all thienopyridines, is a prodrug that requires hepatic metabolism to give origin to its active metabolite that irreversibly inhibits the P2Y12 receptor [24]. In the TRITON-TIMI 38 study (*Trial to Assess Improvement in Therapeutic Outcomes by Optimizing Platelet Inhibition With Prasugrel–Thrombolysis in Myocardial Infarction 38*) 13,608 patients with moderate-to-high-risk ACS with scheduled PCI were assigned to receive prasugrel (a 60-mg loading dose and a 10-mg daily maintenance dose) or clopidogrel (a 300-mg loading dose and a 75-mg daily maintenance dose), for 6–15 months [25]. This trial observed a significant reduction in the rates of the primary end point (composite of CV death, nonfatal MI, or nonfatal stroke) favoring prasugrel (9.9 % vs. 12.1 %; HR = 0.81;

$p < 0.001$) as well as a reduction in the rates of stent thrombosis over a follow-up period of 15 months at the expense of an increased risk of major bleeding in the prasugrel group. Interestingly enough, particular subgroups appeared to have a higher benefit with prasugrel therapy such as patients with STEMI and, importantly, DM patients [26]. Indeed, the reduction of major CV events with prasugrel was higher in DM (12.2 % vs. 17.0 %; HR, 0.70; $p < 0.001$) than non-DM patients (9.2 % vs. 10.6 %; hazard ratio [HR], 0.86; $p = 0.02$). Moreover, a benefit for prasugrel was observed among DM subjects with (14.3 % vs. 22.2 %; HR, 0.63; $p = 0.009$) and without insulin therapy (11.5 % vs. 15.3 %; HR, 0.74; $p = 0.009$) (Fig. 11.2) [26]. These data demonstrate that the more intensive oral antiplatelet therapy provided with prasugrel is of particular benefit to patients with DM.

11.5   Ticagrelor

Ticagrelor, a reversible $P2Y_{12}$ inhibitor, has recently shown to achieve higher inhibition of platelet aggregation than clopidogrel in ACS patients [28]. In patients with DM enrolled in the PLATO study ($n = 4,662$), prasugrel reduced the primary composite endpoint (HR = 0.88; 95 % CI, 0.76–1.03), all-cause mortality (HR = 0.82; 95 % CI, 0.66–1.01), and stent thrombosis (HR = 0.65; 95 % CI, 0.36–1.17) with no increase in major bleeding (HR = 0.95; 95 % CI, 0.81–1.12). Of note such benefit was consistent within the overall cohort and without DM status-by-treatment interactions (Fig. 11.2) [29]. Based on these evidence, current guidelines recommend the use of a $P2Y_{12}$ receptor blocker in patients with DM and ACS for 1 year and in those undergoing PCI (duration depending on stent type). Prasugrel and ticagrelor may be preferred to clopidogrel in patients with PCI and ACS (Table 11.1) [13].

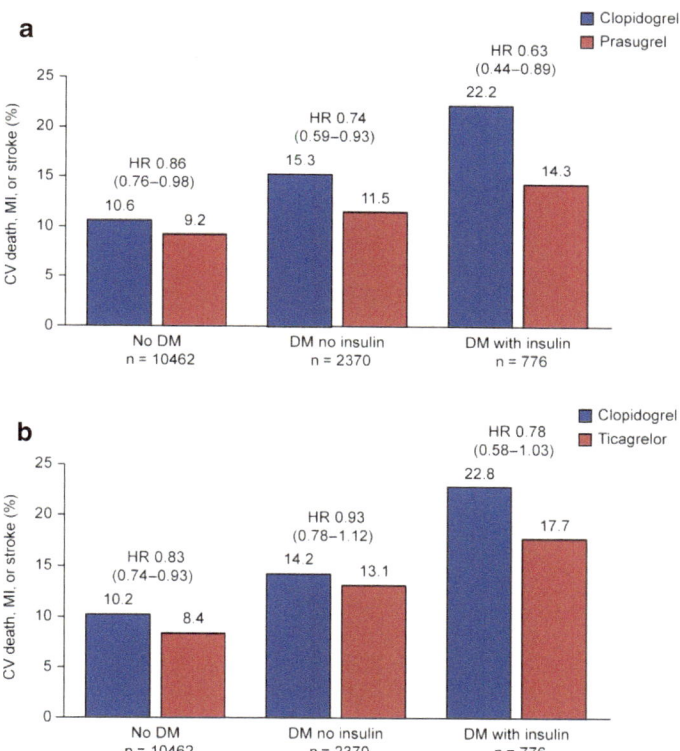

Fig. 11.2 (**a**) Clinical events and relative benefit of prasugrel versus clopidogrel for patients with and without diabetes in the TRITON-TIMI-38 trial. Prasugrel-related benefits appear to be enhanced in diabetic patients, with further benefit observed among those on insulin therapy (Modified from Wiviott et al. [26]). (**b**) Clinical events and relative benefit of ticagrelor versus clopidogrel for patients with and without diabetes in the TRITON-TIMI-38 trial. The absolute benefit of ticagrelor tend to be larger in diabetic patients treated with insulin (Modified from James et al. [27])

Table 11.1 Recent clinical trials showing efficacy of new antiplatelet drugs in patients with diabetes

Trial	Population	Intervention	Outcome	Implications
TRITON-TIMI 38	3,146 subjects with history of DM (776 on insulin)	Prasugrel (60 mg/ 10 mg) vs. clopidogrel (300 mg/75 mg) for 6–15 months	Prasugrel reduced the primary CV end point among non-DM (HR, 0.86; $p=0.02$), and DM patients (HR, 0.70; $p<0.001$)	DM subjects tended to have a greater reduction in ischemic events without an observed increase in major bleeding. These data demonstrate that oral antiplatelet therapy with prasugrel is of particular benefit for patients with DM.
PLATO	4,662 patients with pre-existing DM (1,036 on insulin)	Ticagrelor (180 mg/ 90 mg) vs. clopidogrel (300–600 mg/75 mg)	Ticagrelor reduced the primary composite endpoint (HR, 0.88, 95 % CI: 0.76–1.03), all-cause mortality (HR, 0.82, 95 % CI: 0.66–1.01), and stent thrombosis (HR, 0.65, 95 % CI: 0.36–1.17) with no increase in major bleeding (HR, 0.95, 95 % CI: 0.81–1.12)	As compared to clopidogrel, ticagrelor reduces ischemic events in ACS patients irrespective of DM status and glycemic control, and without an increase in major bleeding events.

| CURRENT-OASIS 7 | 3,844 patients with T2D | Double dose (600/150/75 mg) vs. standard dose (300 mg/75 mg) of clopidogrel | Double dose clopidogrel did not reduce the rate of the primary outcome in the subgroup of DM patients (HR, 0.89 (0.68–1.18), $p=0.43$) | Double-dose clopidogrel regimen was associated with a reduction in CV events and stent thrombosis compared with the standard dose. However, in the subgroup of DM patients no significant effects were observed. Further randomized studies in DM patients are needed to clarify this issue. |

CV cardiovascular, DM diabetes mellitus, T2D type 2 diabetes, HR hazard ratio, CI confidence interval

References

1. Jagroop A, Mikhailidis DP (2012) Platelets and diabetes: A complex association. Platelets. doi:10.3109/09537104.2012.746456
2. Randriamboavonjy V, Fleming I (2012) Platelet function and signaling in diabetes mellitus. Curr Vasc Pharmacol 10:532–538
3. Angiolillo DJ, Roffi M, Fernandez-Ortiz A (2011) Tackling the thrombotic burden in patients with acute coronary syndrome and diabetes mellitus. Expert Rev Cardiovasc Ther 9:697–710
4. Vinik AI, Erbas T, Park TS, Nolan R, Pittenger GL (2001) Platelet dysfunction in type 2 diabetes. Diabetes Care 24:1476–1485
5. Basili S, Pacini G, Guagnano MT, Manigrasso MR, Santilli F, Pettinella C et al (2006) Insulin resistance as a determinant of platelet activation in obese women. J Am Coll Cardiol 48:2531–2538
6. Rocca B, Santilli F, Pitocco D, Mucci L, Petrucci G, Vitacolonna E et al (2012) The recovery of platelet cyclooxygenase activity explains interindividual variability in responsiveness to low-dose aspirin in patients with and without diabetes. J Thromb Haemost 10:1220–1230
7. Preventive Services US (2009) Task Force. Aspirin for the prevention of cardiovascular disease: U.S. Preventive Services Task Force recommendation statement. Ann Intern Med 150:396–404
8. Vandvik PO, Lincoff AM, Gore JM, Gutterman DD, Sonnenberg FA, Alonso-Coello P et al (2012) Primary and secondary prevention of cardiovascular disease: Antithrombotic Therapy and Prevention of Thrombosis, 9th ed: American College of Chest Physicians Evidence-Based Clinical Practice Guidelines. Chest 141:e637S–e668S
9. Baigent C, Blackwell L, Collins R, Emberson J, Godwin J, Peto R et al (2009) Aspirin in the primary and secondary prevention of vascular disease: collaborative meta-analysis of individual participant data from randomised trials. Lancet 373:1849–1860
10. Ogawa H, Nakayama M, Morimoto T, Uemura S, Kanauchi M, Doi N et al (2008) Low-dose aspirin for primary prevention of atherosclerotic events in patients with type 2 diabetes: a randomized controlled trial. JAMA 300:2134–2141
11. Belch J, MacCuish A, Campbell I, Cobbe S, Taylor R, Prescott R et al (2008) The prevention of progression of arterial disease and diabetes (POPADAD) trial: factorial randomised placebo controlled trial of aspirin and antioxidants in patients with diabetes and asymptomatic peripheral arterial disease. BMJ 337:a1840
12. Pignone M, Alberts MJ, Colwell JA, Cushman M, Inzucchi SE, Mukherjee D et al (2010) Aspirin for primary prevention of cardiovascular

events in people with diabetes: a position statement of the American Diabetes Association, a scientific statement of the American Heart Association, and an expert consensus document of the American College of Cardiology Foundation. Circulation 121:2694–2701

13. Ryden L, Grant PJ, Anker SD, Berne C, Cosentino F, Danchin N et al (2013) ESC Guidelines on diabetes, pre-diabetes, and cardiovascular diseases developed in collaboration with the EASD: the Task Force on diabetes, pre-diabetes, and cardiovascular diseases of the European Society of Cardiology (ESC) and developed in collaboration with the European Association for the Study of Diabetes (EASD). Eur Heart J 34:3035–3087

14. Beckman JA, Paneni F, Cosentino F, Creager MA (2013) Diabetes and vascular disease: pathophysiology, clinical consequences, and medical therapy: part II. Eur Heart J 34:2444–2452

15. Patrono C, Andreotti F, Arnesen H, Badimon L, Baigent C, Collet JP et al (2011) Antiplatelet agents for the treatment and prevention of atherothrombosis. Eur Heart J 32:2922–2932

16. Verheugt FW (2015) The role of the cardiologist in the primary prevention of cardiovascular disease with aspirin. J Am Coll Cardiol 65: 122–124

17. Patrono C (2013) Low-dose aspirin in primary prevention: cardioprotection, chemoprevention, both, or neither? Eur Heart J 34:3403–3411

18. American Diabetes Association (2014) Standards of medical care in diabetes–2014. Diabetes Care 37 Suppl 1:S14–S80

19. Arjomand H, Roukoz B, Surabhi SK, Cohen M (2003) Platelets and antiplatelet therapy in patients with diabetes mellitus. J Invasive Cardiol 15:264–269

20. Caprie Steering Committee (1996) A randomised, blinded, trial of clopidogrel versus aspirin in patients at risk of ischaemic events (CAPRIE). CAPRIE Steering Committee. Lancet 348:1329–1339

21. Bhatt DL, Marso SP, Hirsch AT, Ringleb PA, Hacke W, Topol EJ (2002) Amplified benefit of clopidogrel versus aspirin in patients with diabetes mellitus. Am J Cardiol 90:625–628

22. Bhatt DL, Fox KA, Hacke W, Berger PB, Black HR, Boden WE et al (2006) Clopidogrel and aspirin versus aspirin alone for the prevention of atherothrombotic events. N Engl J Med 354:1706–1717

23. Yusuf S, Zhao F, Mehta SR, Chrolavicius S, Tognoni G, Fox KK et al (2001) Effects of clopidogrel in addition to aspirin in patients with acute coronary syndromes without ST-segment elevation. N Engl J Med 345:494–502

24. Fuster V, Farkouh ME (2008) Acute coronary syndromes and diabetes mellitus: a winning ticket for prasugrel. Circulation 118:1607–1608

25. Wiviott SD, Braunwald E, McCabe CH, Horvath I, Keltai M, Herrman JP et al (2008) Intensive oral antiplatelet therapy for reduction of ischaemic events including stent thrombosis in patients with acute coronary syndromes treated with percutaneous coronary intervention and stenting in the TRITON-TIMI 38 trial: a subanalysis of a randomised trial. Lancet 371:1353–1363
26. Wiviott SD, Braunwald E, Angiolillo DJ, Meisel S, Dalby AJ, Verheugt FW et al (2008) Greater clinical benefit of more intensive oral antiplatelet therapy with prasugrel in patients with diabetes mellitus in the trial to assess improvement in therapeutic outcomes by optimizing platelet inhibition with prasugrel-Thrombolysis in Myocardial Infarction 38. Circulation 118:1626–1636
27. James S et al (2010) Ticagrelor vs. clopidogrel in patients with acute coronary syndromes and diabetes: a substudy from the PLATelet inhibition and patient Outcomes (PLATO) trial. Eur Heart J 31:3006–3016
28. Ferreiro JL, Angiolillo DJ (2011) Diabetes and antiplatelet therapy in acute coronary syndrome. Circulation 123:798–813
29. Wallentin L, Becker RC, Budaj A, Cannon CP, Emanuelsson H, Held C et al (2009) Ticagrelor versus clopidogrel in patients with acute coronary syndromes. N Engl J Med 361:1045–1057

Part III
Treatment of Cardiovascular Diseases in Patients with Diabetes

Chapter 12
Coronary Artery Disease

12.1 Medical Therapy vs. Myocardial Revascularization

Epicardial coronary lesions in patients with DM are more extensive and diffuse than non-DM subjects [1]. DM patients also display higher propensity to develop re-stenosis after percutaneous coronary intervention (PCI) and saphenous graft occlusion after coronary artery bypass graft surgery (CABG) and unremitting atherosclerotic progression causing new stenosis [2]. These processes are the result of accelerated atherosclerosis which is mostly triggered by vascular inflammation, endothelial dysfunction, oxidative stress, impaired insulin signaling, and altered lipid metabolism [3]. One of the main evidence gap in the cure of DM is to identify the best revascularization strategy [4]. For example, it remains uncertain whether optimal medical therapy (OMT) is a safe approach for DM patients with stable coronary artery disease (CAD). The *Clinical Outcomes Utilizing Revascularization and Aggressive Drug Evaluation* (COURAGE) trial included 2,287 patients with stable CAD and compared the outcomes of OMT with and without PCI [5]. Over

F. Paneni, F. Cosentino, *Diabetes and Cardiovascular Disease:*
A Guide to Clinical Management, DOI 10.1007/978-3-319-17762-5_12,
© Springer International Publishing Switzerland 2015

a median 4.6 years of follow up, the addition of PCI to OMT did not reduce death and MI as compared to OMT alone, either in the entire cohort or the subgroup with DM. Thus, in stable CAD, patients with DM should be treated with OMT to prevent death and MI, unless an ACS develops. Seven randomized trials have shown that PCI is not superior to OMT for the reduction of major vascular events but improves symptoms and may be applied on an individual basis, should medical therapy fail [6]. The *Bypass Angioplasty Revascularization Investigation 2 Diabetes* (BARI 2D) trial provided similar results [7]. In this trial, 2,368 patients with T2D and CAD were given OMT and randomized to prompt revascularization or expected management. In the revascularization arm, the responsible physician determined the appropriate strategy. Over the course of 5-year follow up, there was no difference in survival between OMT and revascularization arms in total, or by type. In a secondary outcome, patients in the CABG portion of the study who underwent surgery had a significantly lower rate of major CV events (death, MI, or stroke) than those allocated to OMT. This may have resulted because the patients in the CABG arm had more triple vessel coronary artery disease (52.4 % vs. 20.3 %) [3]. Hence, the benefit of CABG over medical therapy seems to be driven by a preference for CABG rather than PCI among patients with more advanced CAD. A further study addressing outcome based on angiographic features showed that the 5-year risk of death, MI or stroke was significantly lower and amplified for those assigned to revascularization when compared to OMT (24.8 % vs. 36.8 %, respectively; $p = 0.005$) [8]. Along the same line of COURAGE and BARI 2D, the MASS-II trial did not show a benefit of initial PCI (angioplasty and BMS only) to OMT in stable CAD [9, 10]. Conversely, revascularization with CABG was associated with significantly fewer MACCE and nonfatal MI both in BARI-2D and MASS-II as compared to OMT alone. Although these studies have shown a comparable outcome with OMT and PCI, some aspects deserve further discussion. COURAGE and BARI-2D utilized mostly balloon angioplasty and BMS. Both these trials were conducted in the preDES era, therefore these data should be interpreted with caution [11]. BARI-2D was limited by a very selected cohort of low-risk patients with only 20.3 % patients having multivessel disease in PCI vs. 52.4 % in CABG. Moreover, mean left ventricular ejection fraction (LVEF) was 57 % in revascularization group, whereas only 17.5 % had LVEF <50 %. Finally, left main disease was excluded and the results could not be generalized to the high-risk DM groups with multivessel disease as in most of the other earlier trials. Further, in COURAGE, there was a 32 % crossover from medical to PCI group (due to ischemia) in an intention to treat trial, and this may have skewed the results against PCI. The level of multidrug compliance achieved was unrealistic in the trial (90 % compliance for triple therapy with aspirin, statin and β blockers) as opposed to 21 % in the real world CRUSADE registry [11, 12]. DES were used in only 2.7 % of the patients (they were introduced in only the last 6 months of the trial). Studies have clearly shown that DES provide significant reduction in clinical and angiographic restenosis albeit without an impact on death and nonfatal MI [13, 14] (Table 12.1).

An important factor which may help cardiologists to choose among OMT or PCI is the burden of myocardial ischemia assessed by positron emission tomography myocardial perfusion imaging (PET-MPI). PET perfusion abnormalities have been shown to provide incremental prognostic value by chi-square analysis in four major studies including 3,897 subjects [15]. Importantly, the presence and extent of ischemic myocardium was able to predict a composite of cardiac death, nonfatal MI, late revascularization, and unstable angina in 685 patients undergoing dipyridamole 82Rb PET MPI [16]. A larger study on 1,432 patients showed that the percentage of ischemic myocardium correlated closely with the risk of cardiac death or nonfatal MI [17]. Patients without ischemia had a 0.7 % annualized event rate, which increased to

Table 12.1 Data from BARI-2D trial comparing optimal medical therapy with myocardial revascularization strategies

Trial	n	MVD (%)	Endpoint	Follow-up	Outcome
Revascularization vs. medical therapy					
BARI-2D 2009	2,368	31	Death	5	Death: 11.7 vs. 12.2 %
					CV death: 5.9 vs. 5.7 %
					MI: 11.5 vs. 14.4 %
					Stroke: 2.6 vs. 2.8 %
CABG vs. medical therapy					
BARI-2D 2009	763	57	Death	5	Death: 13.6 vs. 16.4 %
					CV death: 8.0 vs. 9.0 %
					MI: 10.0 vs. 17.6 %
					Stroke: 1.9 vs. 2.6 %
PCI vs. medical therapy					
BARI-2D 2009	1,605	20	Death	5	Death: 10.8 vs. 10.2 %
					CV death: 5.0 vs. 4.2 %
					MI: 12.3 vs. 12.6 %
					Stroke: 2.9 vs. 2.9 %

MVD multi-vessel disease, *PCI* percutaneous coronary revascularization, *CABG* coronary artery bypass grafting, *CV* cardiovascular

11 % for those with 20 % left ventricular ischemia. Of note, survival in these patients started to be significantly reduced when ischemic myocardium was >10 % [17]. Therefore, quantification of myocardial ischemia may be important to overall decision making in asymptomatic DM patients with CAD (Fig. 12.1).

12.2   PCI vs. CABG

Evidence available so far indicates that surgical revascularization with CABG is the first approach to be considered in DM patients with multivessel disease [12, 18]. Percutaneous revascularization may be indicated in particular cases, especially when anatomy of coronary lesions is favorable and

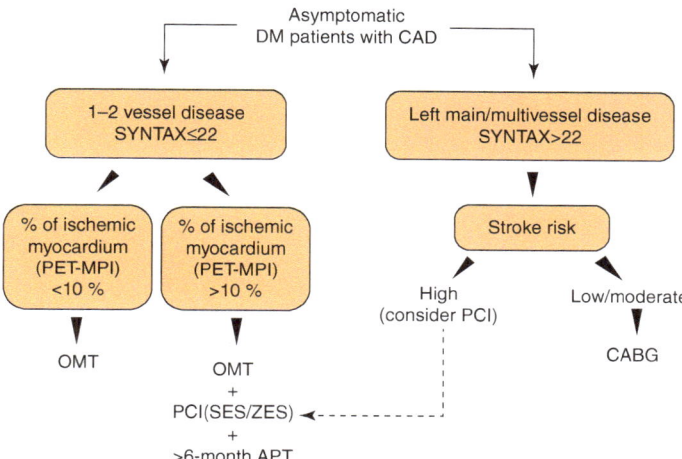

Fig. 12.1 Tentative algorithm for the management of coronary artery disease in asymptomatic patients with diabetes. *DES* drug-eluting stent, *CABG* coronary artery bypass grafting, *PCI* percutaneous coronary intervention, *CAD* coronary artery disease, *OMT* optimal medical therapy; *PET-MPI* positron emission tomography-myocardial perfusion imaging, *APT* antiplatelet therapy

CABG-related risks are too high [12]. The main problem concerning the direct comparison of PCI with CABG derives from the heterogeneity of stents used in different registries and trials. Several authors have claimed that benefit of CABG in many studies was driven by the choice of implanted stents. The BARI registry (*Bypass angioplasty Revascularization Investigation*) has compared 5-year survival in 1,829 DM patients undergoing PCI or CABG. Long term survival was comparable among the two groups (CABG 89.3 % vs. PCI 86.3 %, =0.19); however revascularization procedures were more frequent in PCI-treated (54 %) than CABG (8 %) patients [19]. A sub-analysis of this study including DM patients with multivessel disease showed that PCI was associated with twofold mortality risk as compared to CABG patients (44.3 % vs. 23.6 %, $p < 0.001$) [20]. However, more than 70 % of DM patients received balloon angioplasty in BARI whereas CABG therapy included at last one arterial graft, which is associated with a more favorable prognosis than venous grafts [18]. These aspects might have contributed to CABG-related benefits observed in the BARI population. The 10-year follow up of BARI confirmed that survival was higher in patients receiving surgical as compared to percutaneous revascularization (58 % vs. 45 %, $p = 0.025$) [21]. A more specific comparison of the efficacy and safety of PCI and CABG in patients with DM was performed in the *Coronary Artery Revascularization in Diabetes* (CARDia) trial [22]. This study was launched to better understand whether advances in stent technology could improve CV outcome in DM people. In CARDia, a total of 510 DM patients with multivessel or complex single-vessel coronary disease from 24 centers were randomized to PCI plus stenting (and routine abciximab) or CABG. Among PCI patients, BMS were used initially, but a switch to sirolimus drug-eluting stents was made when these became available. At 1 year of follow-up, the composite rate of death, MI, and stroke was 10.5 % in the CABG group and 13.0 % in the PCI group (HR: 1.25, 95 % CI: 0.75–2.09; $p = 0.39$). However, when CABG patients were compared with the subset of patients who received drug-eluting stents (69 % of patients), the primary outcome rates were 12.4 % and 11.6 % (HR: 0.93, 95 % CI: 0.51–1.71; $p = 0.82$), respectively [22]. These data suggest that PCI may be not inferior to CABG when proper stents are being used for revascularization. Yet, sample size and number of events were not sufficient to draw solid conclusions in this regard. In the SYNTHAX trial, 1,800 patients with three-vessel or left main coronary artery disease were randomized to CABG or PCI with DES (in a 1:1 ratio) [23]. Although appropriate stent choice, the rates of major adverse cardiac or cerebrovascular events at 12 months were significantly higher in the PCI group (17.8 vs. 12.4 % for CABG; $P=0.002$), in large part due to an increased rate of repeat revascularization (13.5 vs. 5.9 %, $P<0.001$). This trial was powered enough to conclude that a noninferiority criteria between PCI and CABG was not met. Along the same line, the FREEDOM trial randomized 1,900 patients – a majority with three-vessel disease – to treatment with CABG or PCI with sirolimus-eluting and paclitaxel-eluting stents [24]. The primary outcome occurred more frequently in the PCI group ($P<0.005$), with a five-year rate of 26.6 %, compared with 18.7 % in the CABG group. The benefit of CABG was driven by differences in both MI ($P<0.001$) and mortality ($P<0.049$). This study confirms that CABG remains the standard of care for patients with three-vessel or left main coronary artery disease [25]. Very recently, a Bayesian network meta-analysis including 40 studies was performed to compare long-term outcomes between the PCI (accounting for the variation in stent choice) and CABG [26]. The primary outcome, a composite of all-cause mortality, nonfatal MI, and stroke, increased with PCI (OR, 1.33 [95 % CI 1.01–1.65]). PCI resulted in increased mortality (OR, 1.44 [95 % CI, 1.05–1.91]), no change in the number of myocardial infarctions (OR, 1.33 [95 % CI, 0.86–1.95]), and fewer strokes (OR, 0.56 [95 % CI, 0.36–0.88]). This analysis confirms that CABG is superior to PCI, regardless to stent choice (Fig. 12.2) [26]. Based on these studies, current recommendations suggest CABG in patients with DM and multivessel or complex (SYNTAX Score >22) CAD to improve survival free from major CV events [12]. By contrast, the indication to PCI is less clear, and less evidence-based. Indeed, PCI is recommended for symptom control, and may be considered as an alternative to CABG in patients with DM at high stroke risk and less complex multivessel CAD (SYNTAX score ≤22) [12]. Whereas CABG-related benefits are clear, the main evidence gap is to identify

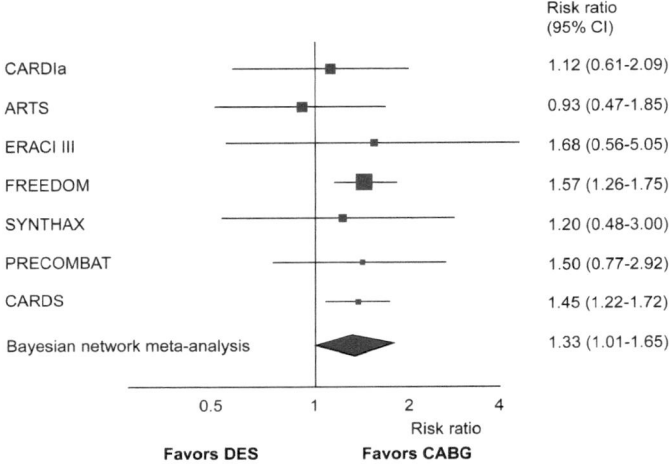

Fig. 12.2 Meta-analysis of randomized controlled trials showing composite end point of all-cause mortality, MI, and stroke in diabetic patients treated with DES versus CABG. *BMS* bare-metal stent, *CABG* coronary artery bypass grafting (Modified from Tu et al. [26])

subjects who may benefit from PCI in current clinical practice (Table 12.2).

12.3   Bare-Metal vs. Drug-Eluting Stents

The DIABETES trial was designed to test the efficacy of sirolimus-eluting stents (SES) compared with standard stents to prevent restenosis in DM patients with de novo lesions in native coronary arteries [27]. One hundred sixty patients were randomized to SES (80 patients; 111 lesions) or standard stent implantation (80 patients; 110 lesions). Over a 9-month follow-up, target-lesion revascularization (31.3 vs. 7.3 %, $P < 0.001$)

Table 12.2 Major randomized controlled trials comparing efficacy of coronary artery bypass grafting (CABG) with percutaneous coronary intervention (PCI) in patients with diabetes

Trial	Stratum	Overall mortality	CV death	Stroke	Revascularization	Nonfatal MI	MACCE	FU (yrs)
ARTS 2005 (n=208)	BMS vs. CABG	13.4 vs. 8.3 (p=0.27)	–	6.3 vs. 7.3 (p=0.79)	42.9 vs. 10.4 (p<0.01)	10.7 vs. 7.3 (p=0.47)	54.5 vs. 25 (p<0.001)	5
BARI 2007 (n=353)	PTCA vs. CABG	54.5 vs. 42.1 (p=0.025)	35.6 vs. 21 (p=0.008)	–	79.7 vs. 18.3 (p<0.001)	58.6 vs. 58.2 (p=0.28)	–	10
CARDIa 2009 (n=502)	BMS/SES vs. CABG	3.2 vs. 3.2 (p=0.97)	–	0.4 vs. 2.8 (p=0.06)	11.8 vs. 2.0 (p<0.001)	9.8 vs. 5.7 (p=0.088)	11.3 vs. 19.3 (p=0.016)	1
SYNTHAX 2009 (n=452)	PES vs. CABG	19.5 vs. 12.9 (p=0.065)	12.7 vs. 6.5 (p=0.034)	3 vs. 4.7 (p=0.34)	35.3 vs. 14.6 (p<0.001)	9.0 vs. 5.4 (p=0.2)	46.5 vs. 29 (p<0.001)	5
FREEDOM 2012 (n=1,900)	DES vs. CABG	16.3 vs. 10.9 (p=0.049)	10.9 vs. 6.8 (p=0.12)	2.4 vs. 5.2 (p=0.03)	–	13.9 vs. 6 (p<0.001)	26.6 vs. 18.7 (p=0.005)	5
VA VARDS 2013 (n=198)	DES vs. CABG	21 vs. 5 (HR 0.3, CI 0.11–0.8)	10.8 vs. 5 (HR 0.53, CI 0.16–1.77)	1.0 vs. 1.2 (HR 1.03, CI 0.06–16.49)	18.9 vs. 19.5 (HR 0.93, CI 0.42–2.07)	6.2 vs. 15 (HR 3.32, CI 1.07–10.3)	–	2

DES drug-eluting stent, *CABG* coronary artery bypass grafting, *CV* cardiovascular, *MACCE* major adverse cardiac and cerebrovascular events, *FU* follow-up, *yrs* years

and major adverse cardiac event rates (36.3 vs. 11.3 %, $P<0.001$) were significantly lower in the sirolimus group. Moreover, stent thrombosis occurred in 2 patients after standard stent implantation whereas this phenomenon was not seen in the sirolimus stent group. The DIABETES was the first randomized study to demonstrate that sirolimus stent implantation is safe and efficacious in reducing both angiographic and clinical parameters of restenosis compared with BMS in patients with DM [27]. Stettler and colleagues performed a meta-analysis including 35 stent trials for a total of 3,852 DM patients [28]. This study revealed a similar efficacy of SES and paclitaxel-eluting stents (PES) in this regard (OR 0.29 for sirolimus; 0.38 for paclitaxel), provided that dual antiplatelet therapy after DES implantation was continued for >6 months. By contrast, DES use is associated with increased CV mortality when antiplatelet therapy is less than 6 months (Table 12.3).

12.4   First vs. Second Generation DES

More recently, new generation DES (everolimus eluting stents, EES) have been tested in randomized trials in patients with and without DM. In the SPIRIT IV trial, EES compared with PES reduced target lesion failure (TLF) in non-DM patients (3.1 % vs. 6.7 %, $p<0.0001$), with significant reductions in MI, stent thrombosis, and target lesion revascularization [29]. In contrast, no difference in TLF (6.4 % vs. 6.9 %, respectively, $p=0.80$) or any of its components was present among DM patients, regardless of insulin use. This study demonstrates that new generation DES are effective in non-DM patients whereas their benefit is comparable to PES in DM people, suggesting that diabetic disease itself may contribute to the observed lack of benefit. Similarly, a substudy of the SORT OUT III trial was not able to show any benefit of second generation DES, endeavor zotarolimus-eluting stent

Table 12.3 Major randomized controlled trials comparing efficacy of drug-eluting stents (DES) versus bare metal stents (BMS), as well as new (EES, ZES) versus old generation DES (SES, PES)

Trial	Stratum	Overall mortality	CV death	Revascularization/ TVF	MI	MACCE	FU
DIABETES 2005 (n=160)	SES vs. BMS	–	–	6.3 vs. 31.3 (p<0.01)	–	10.0 vs. 36.3 (p<0.001)	270 days
DEAR 2012 (n=91)	PEB vs. BMS vs. DES	3.3 vs. 6.5 vs. 6.2 (p=NS)	2.2 vs. 3.3 vs. 2.3 (p=NS)	6.6 vs. 21 vs. 9.4 (*p=0.02; †p=0.77)	3.3 vs. 7.2 vs. 6.2 (p=NS)	13.2 vs. 32.3 vs. 18.6 (*p=0.03; †p=0.29)	1 year
SCORPIUS 2012 (n=190)	SES vs. BMS	21 vs. 21 (p=0.98)	14 vs. 12 (p=0.83)	12 vs. 28 (p<0.005)	8 vs. 9 (p=0.81)	34 vs. 49 (p=0.02)	1 year
SPIRIT IV 2010 (n=1,185)	EES vs. PES	4.1 vs. 4.5 (p=0.76)	3.4 vs. 4 (p=0.62)	3.1 vs. 6.7 (p<0.0001)	2.6 vs. 3.7 (p=0.36)	6.4 vs. 7.1 (p=0.71)	1 year
SORT-OUT III 2011 (n=337)	ZES vs. SES	8.3 vs. 5.4 [HR 1.55 (0.67–3.58)]	3.6 vs. 1.2 [HR 3.00 (0.61–14.9)]	14.2 vs. 3.0 [HR 4.99 (1.90–13.1)]	4.7 vs. 0.6 [(HR 8.09, (1.01–64.7)]	18.3 vs. 4.8 [(HR 4.05, 1.86–8.82)]	18 months

(continued)

Table 12.3 (continued)

Trial	Stratum	Overall mortality	CV death	Revascularization/ TVF	MI	MACCE	FU
ESSENCE-DIABETES II 2013 ($n = 256$)	ZES vs. SES	0 vs. 0.8 ($p = 0.99$)	0 vs. 0	–	0.8 vs. 0.8 ($p = 0.99$)	2.4 vs. 1.6 ($p = 0.68$)	Recruitment was prematurely stopped due to discontinuing production of SES
ENDEAVOR III-IV 2013 ($n = 601$)	ZES vs. SES	7.6 vs. 15.0 ($p = 0.004$)	3.7 vs. 7 ($p = 0.066$)	20.2 vs. 26.9 % ($p = 0.065$)	1.3 vs. 5.1 ($p = 0.011$)	17.7 vs. 26.6 ($p = 0.012$)	5 years Pooled analysis of ENDEAVOR III-IV trials

BMS bare metal stents, *DES* drug-eluting stent, *SES* sirolimus DES, *PES* paclitaxel DES, *EES* everolimus DES, *ZES* zotarolimus DES, *TVF* target vessel failure, *CV* cardiovascular, *MACCE* major adverse cardiac and cerebrovascular events, *MI* myocardial infarction

(ZES) on major adverse cardiac events [30]. In DM patients, use of ZES compared to SES was rather associated with an increased risk of major adverse cardiac events (HR 4.05, 95 % CI 1.86–8.82), MI (HR 8.09, 95 % CI 1.01–64.7), target vessel revascularization (HR 4.99, 95 % CI 1.90–13.1), and target lesion revascularization (HR 11.0, 95 % CI 2.59–47.1). In patients without DM, differences in absolute risk were smaller but similarly favored SES. The authors concluded that implantation of ZES compared to SES is associated with a considerable increased risk of adverse events in patients with DM at 18-month follow-up. In contrast with these results a pooled analysis of the ENDEAVOR III-IV trials including 601 patients with DM showed that TVF rate estimate was numerically lower for ZES, but the difference did not reach statistical significance (20.2 vs. 26.9 %, $P = 0.065$) [31]. The 5-year rate of major adverse cardiac events (17.7 vs. 26.6 %, $P = 0.012$), death (7.6 vs. 15.0 %, $P = 0.004$), and MI (1.3 vs. 5.1 %, $P = 0.011$) were significantly lower for ZES versus other DES, suggesting that ZES have favorable long-term outcomes compared to first-generation DES. Whether second generation DES (ZES and EES) should be preferred to early DES (SES and PES) remains largely controversial. Further randomized studies on a larger number of DM patients are warranted to clarify this issue.

References

1. Tomizawa N, Nojo T, Inoh S, Nakamura S (2015) Difference of coronary artery disease severity, extent and plaque characteristics between patients with hypertension, diabetes mellitus or dyslipidemia. Int J Cardiovasc Imaging 31:205–212
2. Ekezue BF, Laditka SB, Laditka JN, Studnicki J, Blanchette CM (2014) Diabetes complications and adverse health outcomes after coronary revascularization. Diabetes Res Clin Pract 103:530–537

3. Beckman JA, Paneni F, Cosentino F, Creager MA (2013) Diabetes and vascular disease: pathophysiology, clinical consequences, and medical therapy: part II. Eur Heart J 34:2444–2452

4. Paneni F (2014) 2013 ESC/EASD guidelines on the management of diabetes and cardiovascular disease: established knowledge and evidence gaps. Diab Vasc Dis Res 11:5–10

5. Boden WE, O'Rourke RA, Teo KK, Hartigan PM, Maron DJ, Kostuk WJ et al (2007) Optimal medical therapy with or without PCI for stable coronary disease. N Engl J Med 356:1503–1516

6. Kereiakes DJ, Teirstein PS, Sarembock IJ, Holmes DR Jr, Krucoff MW, O'Neill WW et al (2007) The truth and consequences of the COURAGE trial. J Am Coll Cardiol 50:1598–1603

7. Frye RL, August P, Brooks MM, Hardison RM, Kelsey SF, MacGregor JM et al (2009) A randomized trial of therapies for type 2 diabetes and coronary artery disease. N Engl J Med 360:2503–2515

8. Brooks MM, Chaitman BR, Nesto RW, Hardison RM, Feit F, Gersh BJ et al (2012) Clinical and angiographic risk stratification and differential impact on treatment outcomes in the Bypass Angioplasty Revascularization Investigation 2 Diabetes (BARI 2D) trial. Circulation 126:2115–2124

9. Chaitman BR, Hadid M, Laddu AA (2010) Choice of initial medical therapy vs. prompt coronary revascularization in patients with type 2 diabetes and stable ischemic coronary disease with special emphasis on the BARI 2D trial results. Curr Opin Cardiol 25:597–602

10. Silvain J, Vignalou JB, Barthelemy O, Kerneis M, Collet JP, Montalescot G (2014) Coronary revascularization in the diabetic patient. Circulation 130:918–922

11. Fernandez SF, Boden WE (2010) Strategies in stable ischemic heart disease: lessons from the COURAGE and BARI-2D trials. Curr Atheroscler Rep 12:423–431

12. Ryden L, Grant PJ, Anker SD, Berne C, Cosentino F, Danchin N et al (2013) ESC Guidelines on diabetes, pre-diabetes, and cardiovascular diseases developed in collaboration with the EASD: the Task Force on diabetes, pre-diabetes, and cardiovascular diseases of the European Society of Cardiology (ESC) and developed in collaboration with the European Association for the Study of Diabetes (EASD). Eur Heart J 34:3035–3087

13. Babapulle MN, Joseph L, Belisle P, Brophy JM, Eisenberg MJ (2004) A hierarchical Bayesian meta-analysis of randomised clinical trials of drug-eluting stents. Lancet 364:583–591

14. Stone GW, Ellis SG, Cox DA, Hermiller J, O'Shaughnessy C, Mann JT et al (2004) A polymer-based, paclitaxel-eluting stent in patients with coronary artery disease. N Engl J Med 350:221–231

15. Bourque JM, Beller GA (2011) Stress myocardial perfusion imaging for assessing prognosis: an update. JACC Cardiovasc Imaging 4:1305–1319

16. Marwick TH, Shan K, Patel S, Go RT, Lauer MS (1997) Incremental value of rubidium-82 positron emission tomography for prognostic assessment of known or suspected coronary artery disease. Am J Cardiol 80:865–870

17. Dorbala S, Hachamovitch R, Curillova Z, Thomas D, Vangala D, Kwong RY et al (2009) Incremental prognostic value of gated Rb-82 positron emission tomography myocardial perfusion imaging over clinical variables and rest LVEF. JACC Cardiovasc Imaging 2:846–854

18. Kolh P, Windecker S (2014) ESC/EACTS myocardial revascularization guidelines 2014. Eur Heart J 35:3235–3236

19. Influence of diabetes on 5-year mortality and morbidity in a randomized trial comparing CABG and PTCA in patients with multivessel disease: the Bypass Angioplasty Revascularization Investigation (BARI) (1997) Circulation 96:1761–1769

20. Investigators BARI (2000) Seven-year outcome in the Bypass Angioplasty Revascularization Investigation (BARI) by treatment and diabetic status. J Am Coll Cardiol 35:1122–1129

21. Investigators BARI (2007) The final 10-year follow-up results from the BARI randomized trial. J Am Coll Cardiol 49:1600–1606

22. Kapur A, Hall RJ, Malik IS, Qureshi AC, Butts J, de Belder M et al (2010) Randomized comparison of percutaneous coronary intervention with coronary artery bypass grafting in diabetic patients. 1-year results of the CARDia (Coronary Artery Revascularization in Diabetes) trial. J Am Coll Cardiol 55:432–440

23. Serruys PW, Morice MC, Kappetein AP, Colombo A, Holmes DR, Mack MJ et al (2009) Percutaneous coronary intervention versus coronary-artery bypass grafting for severe coronary artery disease. N Engl J Med 360:961–972

24. Farkouh ME, Domanski M, Sleeper LA, Siami FS, Dangas G, Mack M et al (2012) Strategies for multivessel revascularization in patients with diabetes. N Engl J Med 367:2375–2384

25. Farmer JA (2014) Strategies for multivessel revascularization in patients with diabetes: the FREEDOM trial. Curr Atheroscler Rep 16:426

26. Tu B, Rich B, Labos C, Brophy JM (2014) Coronary revascularization in diabetic patients: a systematic review and Bayesian network meta-analysis. Ann Intern Med 161:724–732

27. Sabate M, Jimenez-Quevedo P, Angiolillo DJ, Gomez-Hospital JA, Alfonso F, Hernandez-Antolin R et al (2005) Randomized comparison of sirolimus-eluting stent versus standard stent for percutaneous coronary revascularization in diabetic patients: the diabetes and sirolimus-eluting stent (DIABETES) trial. Circulation 112:2175–2183

28. Stettler C, Allemann S, Wandel S, Kastrati A, Morice MC, Schomig A et al (2008) Drug eluting and bare metal stents in people with and without diabetes: collaborative network meta-analysis. BMJ 337:a1331

29. Kereiakes DJ, Cutlip DE, Applegate RJ, Wang J, Yaqub M, Sood P et al (2010) Outcomes in diabetic and nondiabetic patients treated with everolimus- or paclitaxel-eluting stents: results from the SPIRIT IV clinical trial (Clinical Evaluation of the XIENCE V Everolimus Eluting Coronary Stent System). J Am Coll Cardiol 56:2084–2089

30. Maeng M, Jensen LO, Tilsted HH, Kaltoft A, Kelbaek H, Abildgaard U et al (2011) Outcome of sirolimus-eluting versus zotarolimus-eluting coronary stent implantation in patients with and without diabetes mellitus (a SORT OUT III Substudy). Am J Cardiol 108:1232–1237

31. Vardi M, Burke DA, Bangalore S, Pencina MJ, Mauri L, Kandzari DE et al (2013) Long-term efficacy and safety of Zotarolimus-eluting stent in patients with diabetes mellitus: pooled 5-year results from the ENDEAVOR III and IV trials. Catheter Cardiovasc Interv 82:1031–1038

Chapter 13
Acute Coronary Syndromes

13.1 Prevalence and Prognosis

Diabetic (DM) patients presenting with an acute coronary syndrome (ACS) display increased morbidity and mortality rates as compared to non-DM subjects (Fig. 13.1). Mortality is observed in up to 10 % of ACS patients after 30 days, 13 % at 1 year, and 30 % after 5 years [1]. The relative risk of mortality in the different studies ranges from 1.3 to 5.4 after adjusting for demographic and anthropometric characteristics [2, 3]. International registries confirm that DM patients have a less favorable risk-factor profile, less typical presentation, and longer delay in seeking medical attention [1]. Moreover, they present more frequently with arrhythmias, heart failure, renal dysfunction, and major bleeding. DM patients are treated more often with diuretics and inotropic agents while receiving less antiaggregants (glycoprotein IIb/IIIa and clopidogrel), reperfusion therapies, and insulin as compared to nondiabetics [4].

F. Paneni, F. Cosentino, *Diabetes and Cardiovascular Disease:*
A Guide to Clinical Management, DOI 10.1007/978-3-319-17762-5_13,
© Springer International Publishing Switzerland 2015

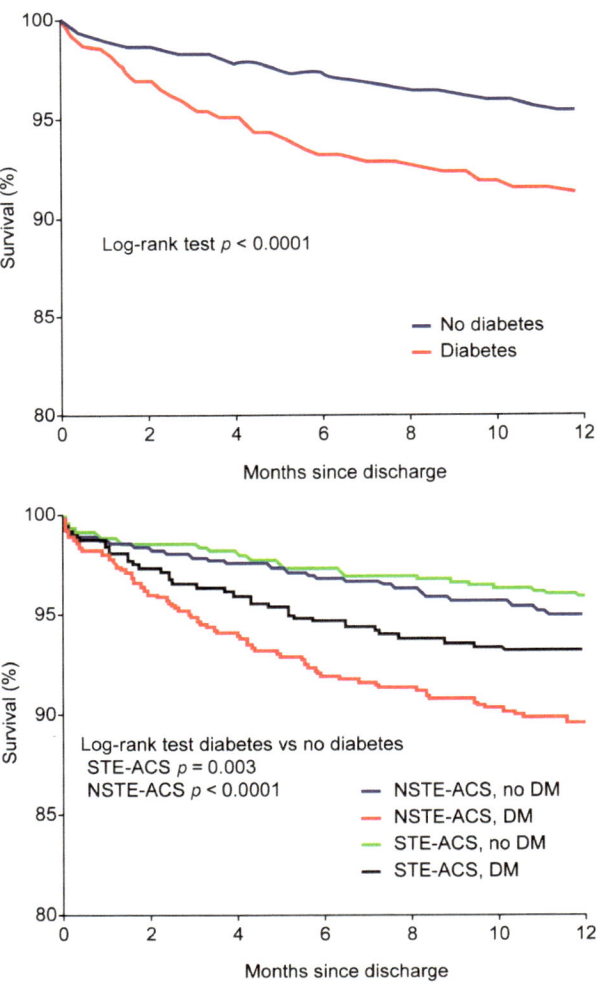

Fig. 13.1 Kaplan-Meier survival curves showing 1-year mortality in patients with and without DM (*upper panel*) and patients with and without DM stratified according to STEMI or non-STEMI (NSTEMI) at presentation (*lower panel*) (Modified with permission from Hasin et al. [4])

13.2 Glycemic Control in Acute Coronary Syndromes

Hyperglycemia is a potent predictor of in-hospital mortality both in ACS patients with and without DM [5, 6]. However, data on the effects of tight glycemic control are inconclusive [7]. The hypothesis that an improved metabolic control may impact on cardiovascular mortality in ACS patients has been postulated in two controlled, randomized clinical trials. The DIGAMI-1 study has enrolled 620 DM patients with ACS randomized to placebo or intensive treatment by insulin-potassium infusion during the first 24 h of ischemia [8]. Such an approach was able to reduce 1-year mortality rate by 30 %, whereas mortality risk reduction was 11 % after 3.4 year follow-up. Based on these findings, the DIGAMI-2 was designed to compare the effectiveness of three treatment strategies: (1) acute insulin-glucose infusion followed by insulin alone; (2) insulin-glucose infusion followed by conventional hypoglycemic treatment; and (3) conventional therapy [9]. This approach is supported by the notion that insulin-glucose administered in the acute phase may rapidly provide a metabolic substrate to the ischemic heart thereby avoiding myocardial FFA oxidation. Moreover, acute insulin infusion has shown to improve platelet functionality, lipid abnormalities, and to reduce PAI-1 activity, thus favoring spontaneous fibrinolysis [10]. The DIGAMI-2 trial, conducted on 1253 DM patients, did not show any difference among treatment arms, indicating that intensive metabolic control by insulin-glucose infusion followed by insulin was not superior to conventional therapy [9]. However, the metabolic control at baseline was much worse than the one observed in DIGAMI-1 and most of patients did not reach an optimal glycemic control. A meta-analysis including several randomized studies on glucose-insulin-potassium (GIK) treatment in ACS has shown a potential benefit of this strategy, with a reduction of mortality rate of 28 % [11]. By contrast, the CREATE-ECLA study which randomized more than 20,000 patients with ST elevation myocardial infarction (STEMI) to GIK therapy did not show any reduction of death, cardiac arrest, and cardiogenic shock [12]. However, it should be noted that only 18 % of recruited patients were diabetic – therefore it is difficult to draw any specific conclusion on this population. Based on these studies, DM patients with ACS may receive an intensive strategy if hyperglycemia is significant (>180 mg/dl) [13]. By contrast, in the presence of comorbidities which increase the risk of hypoglycemia, metabolic control should not be strict to avoid severe complications including mortality [13]. As of today, insulin infusion remains the gold standard to cure diabetic patients with ACS.

13.3   Antithrombotic Therapy

Current evidence suggest that there is no clear indication to adopt different antithrombotic regimens in DM as compared to non-DM patients [7]. In the PLATO trial, ticagrelor equally reduced the rate of ischemic events both in ACS patients with and without DM [14]. Ticagrelor-related benefits were indeed independent of diabetic status and glycemic control, without an increase in major bleeding. An exception is represented by prasugrel which has shown to be superior to clopidogrel, particularly in patients with DM [15, 16]. Indeed, the TRITON-TIMI 38 trial showed that the reduction of major CV events with prasugrel was higher in DM (12.2 % vs. 17.0 %; HR, 0.70; $P<0.001$) than non-DM patients (9.2 % vs. 10.6 %; HR, 0.86; $P=0.02$) [17]. Moreover, the benefit for prasugrel was observed among DM subjects with (14.3 % vs. 22.2 %; HR, 0.63; $P=0.009$) and without insulin therapy (11.5 % vs. 15.3 %; HR, 0.74; $P=0.009$). These data indicate that prasugrel may be considered as a first-line platelet inhibitor in ACS. The use of Gp IIb/IIIa inhibitors does not seem to be supported by current evidence, except for high-risk patients. Previous trials performed without concomitant use of thienopyridines have shown a favorable impact on outcome in DM patients, as confirmed by a meta-analysis [18, 19]. However, the fact that these trials did not use regimens of high clopidogrel loading dose, which are associated with more potent antiplatelet effects and have become the standard of care in clinical practice, but instead used ticlopidine or standard-dose clopidogrel has led to questions about validity of these data in today's practice [19]. The EARLY-ACS trial showed that administration of eptifibatide 12 h or more before angiography in 9,492 NSTEMI patients was not superior to its provisional use after PCI [20]. Early use of eptifibatide was associated with an increased risk of non-life-threatening bleeding and need for transfusion. However, the efficacy of Gp IIb/IIIa inhibitors correlates directly with severity and risk of ACS. Therefore, the risk-benefit ratio should be always assessed in an individualized manner [19]. The ISAR-REACT 2 trial showed a significant reduction in the risk of adverse events with abciximab treatment compared with placebo in patients with high-risk ACS undergoing PCI after pretreatment with 600 mg clopidogrel [21]. Collectively, DM patients with NSTEMI and high troponin release should be treated with Gp IIb/IIIa inhibitors, if bleeding risk is acceptable [22]. The main problem related to this class of drugs is the hemorrhagic risk which may significantly affect the prognosis of ACS patients [19]. In STEMI patients the benefits of Gp IIb/IIIa inhibitors are controversial. Only a few studies have been conducted in the DM population with conflicting results. A meta-analysis of 16 randomized trials including 10,085 patients showed that Gp IIb-IIIa inhibitors did not reduce 30-day mortality (2.8 vs. 2.9 %, $P=0.75$) or re-infarction (1.5 vs. 1.9 %, $P=0.22$), but were associated with higher risk of major bleeding complications (4.1 vs. 2.7 %, $P=0.0004$) [23]. However, high-risk ACS were associated with benefits in terms of death ($P=0.008$) but not re-infarction ($P=0.25$). In contrast, the *Controlled Abciximab and Device Investigation to Lower Late Angioplasty Combinations* (CADILLAC) trial conducted in low-risk ACS patients with DM (n=346) did not find a benefit in terms of death, reinfarction, or stroke with the use of abciximab after balloon angioplasty or stenting [24].

13.4   Anticoagulants

Available evidence indicates that anticoagulation is effective in addition to platelet inhibition and that the combination of the two is more effective than either treatment alone [22]. Fondaparinux, an indirect factor Xa inhibitor, has shown to be not inferior to low weight molecular heparin (LWMH) in reducing the risk of ischemic events. PENTUA and OASIS-5 and 6 trials have clearly demonstrated that the major advantage of fondaparinux is the highest safety profile (low risk of major bleeding) with a consistent reduction of short- and long-term morbidity and mortality [25, 26]. Very recently, a prospective registry including 14,791 patients treated with fondaparinux and 25,825 with low molecular weight heparin (LMWH) showed that the former was associated with significantly less in-hospital bleeding events (adjusted OR, 0.54; 95 % CI, 0.42–0.70) while reduction of CV outcome at 30 and 180 days was comparable among the two groups [27]. Available evidence suggest that fondaparinux should be considered as a first-line anticoagulant in ACS patients. Similarly, a subgroup analysis of the ACUITY-TRIAL performed on the DM cohort (n=3852) showed that monotherapy with the direct thrombin inhibitor bivalirudin was associated with a similar rate of composite ischemia (death, MI, or unplanned ischemic revascularization) compared with Gp IIb/IIIa plus heparin (7.9 % vs. 8.9 %; P=0.39) and a lower rate of major bleedings (3.7 % vs. 7.1 %; P<0.001), resulting in fewer net adverse clinical outcomes (10.9 % vs. 13.8 %; P=0.02). This reduction of ischemic risk is of special importance because DM is a predictor of bleeding complications in patients with ACS and/or PCI [28].

References

1. Sanon S, Patel R, Eshelbrenner C, Sanon VP, Alhaddad M, Oliveros R et al (2012) Acute coronary syndrome in patients with diabetes mellitus: perspectives of an interventional cardiologist. Am J Cardiol 110: 13B–23B

2. Katz P, Leiter LA, Mellbin L, Ryden L (2014) The clinical burden of type 2 diabetes in patients with acute coronary syndromes: prognosis and implications for short- and long-term management. Diab Vasc Dis Res 11:395–409

3. Yeh RW, Sidney S, Chandra M, Sorel M, Selby JV, Go AS (2010) Population trends in the incidence and outcomes of acute myocardial infarction. N Engl J Med 362:2155–2165

4. Hasin T, Hochadel M, Gitt AK, Behar S, Bueno H, Hasin Y (2009) Comparison of treatment and outcome of acute coronary syndrome in patients with versus patients without diabetes mellitus. Am J Cardiol 103:772–778

5. O'Neill BJ, Mann UM, Gupta M, Verma S, Leiter LA (2013) Survey of diabetes care in patients presenting with acute coronary syndromes in Canada. Can J Cardiol 29:1134–1137

6. Mellbin LG, Malmberg K, Ryden L, Wedel H, Vestberg D, Lind M (2013) The relationship between glycaemic variability and cardiovascular complications in patients with acute myocardial infarction and type 2 diabetes: a report from the DIGAMI 2 trial. Eur Heart J 34: 374–379

7. Ryden L, Grant PJ, Anker SD, Berne C, Cosentino F, Danchin N et al (2013) ESC Guidelines on diabetes, pre-diabetes, and cardiovascular diseases developed in collaboration with the EASD: the Task Force on diabetes, pre-diabetes, and cardiovascular diseases of the European Society of Cardiology (ESC) and developed in collaboration with the European Association for the Study of Diabetes (EASD). Eur Heart J 34:3035–3087

8. Malmberg K, Ryden L, Efendic S, Herlitz J, Nicol P, Waldenstrom A et al (1995) Randomized trial of insulin-glucose infusion followed by subcutaneous insulin treatment in diabetic patients with acute myocardial infarction (DIGAMI study): effects on mortality at 1 year. J Am Coll Cardiol 26:57–65

9. Malmberg K, Ryden L, Wedel H, Birkeland K, Bootsma A, Dickstein K et al (2005) Intense metabolic control by means of insulin in patients with diabetes mellitus and acute myocardial infarction (DIGAMI 2): effects on mortality and morbidity. Eur Heart J 26:650–661

10. Ferreiro JL, Cequier AR, Angiolillo DJ (2010) Oral antiplatelet therapy in patients with diabetes mellitus and acute coronary syndromes. Trends Cardiovasc Med 20:211–217

11. Zhao YT, Weng CL, Chen ML, Li KB, Ge YG, Lin XM et al (2010) Comparison of glucose-insulin-potassium and insulin-glucose as adjunctive therapy in acute myocardial infarction: a contemporary meta-analysis of randomised controlled trials. Heart 96:1622–1626

12. Mehta SR, Yusuf S, Diaz R, Zhu J, Pais P, Xavier D et al (2005) Effect of glucose-insulin-potassium infusion on mortality in patients with acute ST-segment elevation myocardial infarction: the CREATE-ECLA randomized controlled trial. JAMA 293:437–446

13. American Diabetes Association (2014) Standards of medical care in diabetes – 2014. Diabetes Care 37(Suppl 1):S14–S80

14. James S, Angiolillo DJ, Cornel JH, Erlinge D, Husted S, Kontny F et al (2010) Ticagrelor vs. clopidogrel in patients with acute coronary syndromes and diabetes: a substudy from the PLATelet inhibition and patient Outcomes (PLATO) trial. Eur Heart J 31:3006–3016

15. Patti G, Proscia C, Di Sciascio G (2014) Antiplatelet therapy in patients with diabetes mellitus and acute coronary syndrome. Circ J 78:33–41

16. Alexopoulos D, Xanthopoulou I, Mavronasiou E, Stavrou K, Siapika A, Tsoni E et al (2013) Randomized assessment of ticagrelor versus prasugrel antiplatelet effects in patients with diabetes. Diabetes Care 36:2211–2216

17. Wiviott SD, Braunwald E, Angiolillo DJ, Meisel S, Dalby AJ, Verheugt FW et al (2008) Greater clinical benefit of more intensive oral anti-platelet therapy with prasugrel in patients with diabetes mellitus in the trial to assess improvement in therapeutic outcomes by optimizing platelet inhibition with prasugrel-Thrombolysis in Myocardial Infarction 38. Circulation 118:1626–1636

18. Roffi M, Chew DP, Mukherjee D, Bhatt DL, White JA, Heeschen C et al (2001) Platelet glycoprotein IIb/IIIa inhibitors reduce mortality in diabetic patients with non-ST-segment-elevation acute coronary syndromes. Circulation 104:2767–2771

19. Ferreiro JL, Angiolillo DJ (2011) Diabetes and antiplatelet therapy in acute coronary syndrome. Circulation 123:798–813

20. Giugliano RP, White JA, Bode C, Armstrong PW, Montalescot G, Lewis BS et al (2009) Early versus delayed, provisional eptifibatide in acute coronary syndromes. N Engl J Med 360:2176–2190

21. Kastrati A, Mehilli J, Neumann FJ, Dotzer F, ten Berg J, Bollwein H et al (2006) Abciximab in patients with acute coronary syndromes undergoing percutaneous coronary intervention after clopidogrel pretreatment: the ISAR-REACT 2 randomized trial. JAMA 295:1531–1538

22. Hamm CW, Bassand JP, Agewall S, Bax J, Boersma E, Bueno H et al (2011) ESC Guidelines for the management of acute coronary syn-

dromes in patients presenting without persistent ST-segment elevation: the Task Force for the management of acute coronary syndromes (ACS) in patients presenting without persistent ST-segment elevation of the European Society of Cardiology (ESC). Eur Heart J 32:2999–3054

23. Boersma E, Harrington RA, Moliterno DJ, White H, Theroux P, Van de Werf F et al (2002) Platelet glycoprotein IIb/IIIa inhibitors in acute coronary syndromes: a meta-analysis of all major randomised clinical trials. Lancet 359:189–198

24. Stone GW, Grines CL, Cox DA, Garcia E, Tcheng JE, Griffin JJ et al (2002) Comparison of angioplasty with stenting, with or without abciximab, in acute myocardial infarction. N Engl J Med 346:957–966

25. Simoons ML, Bobbink IW, Boland J, Gardien M, Klootwijk P, Lensing AW et al (2004) A dose-finding study of fondaparinux in patients with non-ST-segment elevation acute coronary syndromes: the Pentasaccharide in Unstable Angina (PENTUA) Study. J Am Coll Cardiol 43:2183–2190

26. Yusuf S, Mehta SR, Chrolavicius S, Afzal R, Pogue J, Granger CB et al (2006) Effects of fondaparinux on mortality and reinfarction in patients with acute ST-segment elevation myocardial infarction: the OASIS-6 randomized trial. JAMA 295:1519–1530

27. Szummer K, Oldgren J, Lindhagen L, Carrero JJ, Evans M, Spaak J et al (2015) Association between the use of fondaparinux vs low-molecular-weight heparin and clinical outcomes in patients with non-ST-segment elevation myocardial infarction. JAMA 313:707–716

28. Stone GW, McLaurin BT, Cox DA, Bertrand ME, Lincoff AM, Moses JW et al (2006) Bivalirudin for patients with acute coronary syndromes. N Engl J Med 355:2203–2216

Chapter 14
Heart Failure

14.1 Prognosis of Heart Failure in Patients with Diabetes

Epidemiological analyses have clearly outlined the association between heart failure (HF) and diabetes (DM) [1]. HF patients with concomitant DM have a further increase in morbidity and mortality due to coexistence of several mechanisms including disturbed neurohormonal axis as well as structural and functional abnormalities occurring in the diabetic myocardium [2]. About one fifth of patients with chronic HF has DM, and such prevalence reaches 40 % for patients with worsening HF [3, 4]. T2D individuals are at increased risk for both HF with preserved (HFPEF) and reduced (HFREF) ejection fraction. Notably, prospective analyses have shown that the prognosis of HFPEF is comparable to the one reported for HFREF patients, with a 50–60 % mortality rate after 5 years [5, 6]. Recent data show that diabetic HFPEF patients display increased HF hospitalization or HF death as compared to non-DM subjects (30.9 % vs. 19.0 %, respectively), with an estimated 68 % increased risk after adjusting for relevant confounders (adjusted HR 1.68, 95 % confidence interval 1.26–2.25, p <0.001) [7]. Another important aspect to be

F. Paneni, F. Cosentino, *Diabetes and Cardiovascular Disease:*
A Guide to Clinical Management, DOI 10.1007/978-3-319-17762-5_14,
© Springer International Publishing Switzerland 2015

considered is that the prognosis of DM patients with HF remains worse even though these patients are receiving care that is similar to non-DM people [8]. This may be explained by the fact that in DM patients, hyperglycemia and insulin resistance may significantly amplify microvascular disease, defects of intracellular calcium handling as well as reduced myocardial lipid uptake leading to metabolic disturbances, mitochondrial insufficiency, and severe myocyte dysfunction [2]. Beside, patients hospitalized for HF are older, have higher systolic blood pressure values, and have renal dysfunction [4].

14.2   Pharmacological Therapy

Post hoc analyses of different trials have shown that DM patients have responses similar to those without DM [3]. This is particularly true among outpatients with stable HF. By contrast, the efficacy of HF medication in hospitalized DM patients seems to be hampered by the presence of different comorbidities clustering in patients with DM. Indeed, HF-related mortality remains high despite the implementation of guideline-recommended treatments [9].

14.2.1   RAAS Blockade

Randomized studies have reported unequivocal benefits of RAAS inhibition in DM patients with HF (Table 14.1). The SOLVD trial has demonstrated that the addition of the ACE-inhibitor enalapril to conventional therapy significantly reduced mortality and hospitalizations in patients with chronic congestive HF and low EF, and these benefits were reported to be consistent in the subgroup of patients with DM [10]. A retrospective analysis performed on high-risk HF patients in the *Assessment of Treatment with Lisinopril And Survival* (ATLAS) trial showed that DM patients had a beneficial response to high-dose therapy which was comparable to the one observed in non-DM [11]. Angiotensin receptor blockers also represent a valid alternative to ACE-inhibitors. Subgroup analyses of CHARM and Val-HeFT trials showed that the ARBs candestartan and valsartan were associated with consistent risk reductions of CV death or HF hospitalization in DM patients [12, 13]. Similar findings were reported for the aldosterone antagonist eplerenone, which in the EPHESUS trial showed a beneficial effect on CV morbidity and mortality in postacute MI patients with LVEF ≤40 % [14]. However, none of these three sub-analyses was able to achieve statistical significance, likely due to small sample size not powered enough to detect this effect (Table 14.1). The use of spironolactone significantly reduced all-cause mortality in DM (HR 0.70, CI 0.52–0.94) as well as in non-DM patients (HR 0.70, CI 0.60–0.82) with LVEF ≤35 % and NYHA class III–IV [15]. More recent evidence has suggested that Aliskiren, a first-class direct renin inhibitor, might represent a promising therapeutic approach in diabetic with HF. However, in the ASTRONAUT trial, which included 41 % of DM patients, the use of aliskiren in addition to standard therapy did not reduce CV death or HF rehospitalization at 6 months or 12 months after discharge [16]. By contrast, aliskiren increased the rates of hyperkalemia, hypotension, and renal dysfunction [16]. Based on these evidence, ACE-inhibitors are the first choice in DM patients with HFPEF or HFREF to prevent hospitalization and mortality [17]. ARBs are an alternative to ACE-inhibitors when these latter drugs are not tolerated. Current guidelines recommend an aldosterone antagonist for all patients with persisting HF symptoms (NYHA class II–IV) and LVEF ≤35 % despite treatment with an ACE-inhibitor or an ARB [18]. The results of the ASTRONAUT trial do not support the use of aliskiren in this setting [16].

Table 14.1 Major clinical trials in heart failure patients with and without diabetes

Trial	Population	Primary outcome	Treatment	Relative risk	FU (months)
ACE-inhibitors					
SOLVD	HF with EF<35 %	Mortality and hospitalization for worsening HF	Enalapril vs. placebo	0.84 (0.74–0.95) in non-DM vs. 1.01 (0.85–1.21) in DM	41.4
ATLAS	High-risk HF patients	All-cause mortality	Lisinopril high dose vs. lisinopril low-dose	RR reduced by 6 % and 14 % in non-DM and DM, respectively	46
TRACE	MI survivors EF<35 %	All-cause mortality	Trandalapril vs. placebo	0.82 (0.69–0.97) in non-DM vs. 0.64 (0.45–0.91) in DM	26
SAVE	MI survivors EF ≤ 40 %	CV mortality	Captopril vs. placebo	0.82 (0.68–0.99) in non-DM vs. 0.89 (0.68–1.16) in DM	42

ARBs

CHARM	NYHA functional class II–IV EF<40 %	CV death or hospitalization for HF	Candesartan vs. placebo	RR not significant in non-DM vs. DM	40
Val-HeFT	NYHA functional class II–IV	CV mortality and morbidity	Valsartan vs. placebo	RR not significant in non-DM vs. DM	23
Aliskiren					
ASTRONAUT	Stable hospitalized HF	CV death or HF hospitalization	Aliskiren vs. placebo	0.80 (0.64–0.99) in non-DM vs. 1.16 (0.91–1.47) in DM	11.3
LCZ696					
PARADIGM	NYHA functional class II–IV EF<40 %	CV death and hospitalization for HF	LCZ696 vs. enalapril	Significant HR reduction in non-DM and DM patients	27
AA					
EPHESUS	Postacute MI with EF≤40 %	Mortality and CV morbidity	Eplerenone vs. placebo	Significant RR reduction in non-DM and DM patients	16

(continued)

Table 14.1 (continued)

Trial	Population	Primary outcome	Treatment	Relative risk	FU (months)
RALES	NYHA functional class III–IV EF<35 %	All-cause mortality	Spironolactone vs. placebo	0.70 (0.60–0.82) in non-DM vs. 0.70 (0.52–0.94) in DM	24
Beta-blockers					
MERIT-HF	NYHA functional class III–IV EF<40 %	Risk of hospitalization for HF	Metoprolol vs. placebo	RR reduced by 35 % and 37 % in non-DM and DM pts, respectively	12
CIBIS II	NYHA functional class III–IV EF<35 %	All-cause mortality	Bisoprolol vs. placebo	0.66 (0.58–0.81) in no DM vs. 0.81 (0.51–1.28) in DM	16

| COPERNICUS | NYHA functional class IV EF<25 % | All-cause mortality or hospitalization for HF | Carvedilol vs. placebo | 0.67 (0.52–0.85) in non-DM vs. 0.68 (0.47–1.00) in DM | 10.4 |
| COMET | NYHA functional class III–IV EF<35 % | All-cause mortality | Metoprolol vs. carvedilol | Carvedilol reduced all-cause mortality across non-DM and DM subgroups | 58 |

CI confidence interval, *CV* cardiovascular, *DM* diabetes mellitus, *EF* ejection fraction, *HR* hazard ratio, *MI* myocardial infarction, *NYHA* New York Heart Association, *FU* follow-up

14.2.2 Neprilysin Inhibition

Neprilysin, a neutral endopeptidase, degrades several endoge-
nous vasoactive peptides, including natriuretic peptides, brady-
kinin, and adrenomedullin [19]. Inhibition of neprilysin
increases the levels of these substances, countering the neurohormonal overactivation that contributes to vasoconstriction,
sodium retention, and maladaptive remodeling [20]. Combined
inhibition of RAAS and neprilysin had effects that were superior to those of either approach alone in experimental studies
[20]. The recent PARADIGM trial tested the efficacy of the
combination neprilysin inhibitor sacubitril (AHU377) with the
ARB valsartan (LCZ696) as compared with enalapril in patients
with HF [21]. This study was stopped early, according to prespecified rules, after a median follow-up of 27 months, because
the boundary for an overwhelming benefit with LCZ696 versus
enalapril. Indeed, LCZ696 treatment was associated with a significant reduction of death from CV causes or hospitalization
for HF (hazard ratio, 0.80; 95 % CI, 0.71–0.89; $p < 0.001$) [21].
As compared with enalapril, LCZ696 also reduced the risk of
HF hospitalization by 21 % ($p < 0.001$), decreased symptoms
and physical limitations ($p = 0.001$). Notably, these benefits
were consistent in the subgroup of 2,907 DM patients. Neprilysin
inhibition may undoubtedly represent a novel strategy to combat
HF in patients with and without DM [20].

14.2.3 Beta-blockers

Beta-blockers have shown to reduce CV mortality in DM and
non-DM patients with HF. The efficacy of metoprolol, bisoprolol, and carvedilol has been demonstrated in MERIT-HF
[22], CIBIS II [23], and COPERNICUS [24] trials. However,

as observed for RAAS blockers, sub-analyses of these trials including DM subjects showed substantial reduction of HF-related mortality and hospitalization (37 % in MERIT-HF, 19 % in CIBIS II, and 32 % in COPERNICUS), but in the absence of statistical significance [4] (Table 14.1). However, pooling mortality data from CIBIS II, MERIT-HF, and COPERNICUS showed similar survival benefits in patients with [0.76 (95 % CI 0.60–0.96)] and without DM [0.64 (95 % CI 0.56–0.73)] [22]. The main concerns related to the use of beta-blockers in DM are due to the fact that these drugs impair insulin sensitivity and blunt symptoms of hypoglycemia [18]. This particularly applies to non selective beta-blockers such as propanolol [18]. In this regard, the COMET trial has shown that the combined α- and $-\beta$ blocker carvedilol was associated with more favorable metabolic profile as well as with lower incidence of prolonged hypoglycemia [25]. Beta-blockers are recommended in addition to RAAS blockade in DM patients with systolic and diastolic HF to reduce mortality and hospitalization [18]. Carvediol is particularly indicated in patients with poor glycemic status and high risk of hypoglycemia [18].

14.2.4 Diuretics

DM patients are over-treated with diuretics and this worsens their metabolic status with implications on mid-term morbidity [4]. Thiazide and loop diuretics are indeed associated with poor glucose metabolism, an association which is stronger with the formers. However, diuretics remain very useful drugs especially in DM patients with fluid retention and dyspnea, regardless of EF [17]. In general, loop diuretics should be preferred to thiazide diuretics. There is no evidence that diuretics are more effective in DM than non-DM patients with HF.

14.3   Glycemic Control and Risk of Heart Failure

Several studies have shown that poor glycemic control, as indicated by glycated hemoglobin levels, is associated with an increased risk of HF [26]. A recent meta-analysis including seven randomized controlled trials with a total of 37,229 patients showed that the risk of HF-related events did not differ significantly between intensive glycemic control and standard treatment (OR 1.20, 95 % CI 0.96–1.48), but the effect estimate was highly heterogeneous (Fig. 14.1) [27]. Indeed, among the four trials that had a high rate of thiazolidinediones use (i.e., PROactive, ACCORD, VADT, and RECORD), the risk of HF was elevated in individuals randomized to intensive blood glucose control. On the other hand, among the remaining three trials (i.e., UKPDS, ADVANCE, and VA-CSDM), the risk ratio was close to null with a wide CI, highlighting the limitedness of the available data (risk ratio 0.96, 95 % CI 0.81–1.13) [28]. Hence, it is difficult to conclude that hyperglycemia may not be relevant in HF patients and further studies are needed to clarify this important issue. In contrast with this meta-analysis, an earlier cohort study including 25,958 men and 22,900 women with T2D demonstrated that each 1 % increase in HbA_{1c} was associated with an 8 % increased risk of HF (95 % CI 5–2 %) [29]. In this study, an $HbA_{1c} \geq 10$, relative to $HbA_{1c} < 10$ was associated with 1.56-fold (95 % CI 1.26–1.93) greater risk of HF [29]. Similarly, in the Reykjavik Study, a linear and independent relationship between increasing fasting plasma glucose and the development of HF was observed [30]. More recently, in a clinical trial cohort of 531,546 subjects at high CV risk followed-up

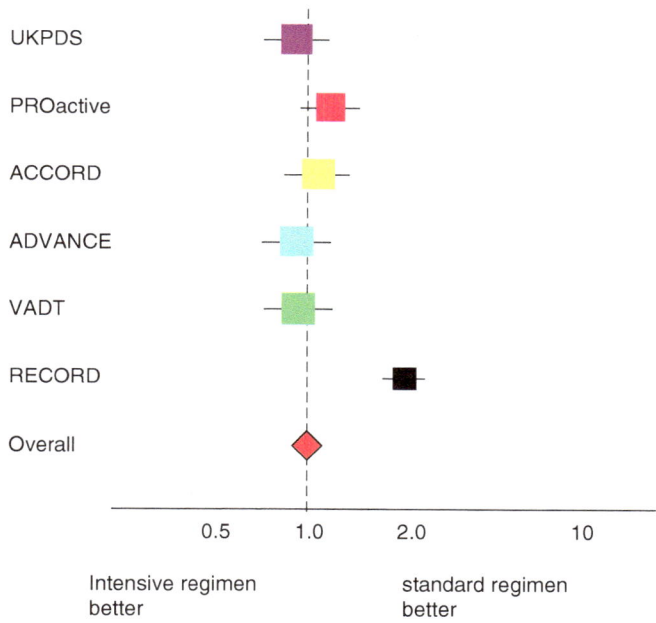

Fig. 14.1 Probability of HF-related events with intensive glucose-lowering versus standard treatment. The size of the markers (*squares*) is approximately proportional to the statistical weight of each trial (Modified from Castagno et al. [27])

for a mean of 2.4 years, Held et al. showed that dysglycemia was an independent predictor of hospitalization for HF regardless of DM status [31]. Collectively, these data suggest that: (1) glycemic burden may be important for HF occurrence and hospitalization, and (2) choice of glucose lowering drugs may affect HF risk in DM patients. Table 14.2 summarizes the effects of various glucose-lowering drugs in DM patients with HF.

Table 14.2 Effect of glucose lowering drugs on the risk of heart failure in patients with diabetes

Glucose-lowering drug	Effects on heart failure
Metformin	Metformin reduces mortality rates in DM with HF [OR 0.65 (0.48–0.87)], even in combination with other agents [OR 0.72 (0.59–0.90)]
	Recent evidence suggests that metformin does not increase the risk of lactic acidosis
Sulfonylureas	Observational studies do not support a relationship between sulfonylureas and HF mortality
Thiazolidinediones	TZD have shown to induce sodium retention and plasma volume expansion, and thus worsening HF
	TZD largely increase incident HF and HF-related hospitalizations
	These drugs should not be used in DM patients with HF
GLP-1 agonists	Cohort studies suggest that GLP-1 agents are associated with reduced risk of HF hospitalization (aHR, 0.51, 0.34–0.77; p =0.002), all-cause hospitalization (aHR 0.54, 95 % CI 0.38–0.74; p =0.001), and death (aHR 0.31, 95 % CI 0.18–0.53; p = .001)
	The ongoing FIGHT trial will clarify whether treatment with liraglutide affect time to death, (2) time to HF hospitalization, and (3) time-averaged proportional change in NT-proBNP in DM patients with advanced HF
DPP-4 inhibitors	Sitagliptin use is not associated with an increased risk of all-cause hospitalizations or death, but was associated with an increased risk of HF-related hospitalizations among 7,620 patients with diabetes and pre-existing HF
	Two recent meta-analyses showed that long-term treatment with DPP-4 is associated with increased risk of HF

Table 14.2 (continued)

Glucose-lowering drug	Effects on heart failure
Insulin	The ORIGIN trial has recently shown that insulin glargine does not affect HF hospitalization and HF-related death after 6.2 years follow-up

DM diabetes mellitus, *HF* heart failure, *TZD* thiazolidinediones, *OR* odds ratio, *aHR* adjusted hazard ratio

References

1. Nichols GA, Gullion CM, Koro CE, Ephross SA, Brown JB (2004) The incidence of congestive heart failure in type 2 diabetes: an update. Diabetes Care 27:1879–1884
2. Boudina S, Abel ED (2007) Diabetic cardiomyopathy revisited. Circulation 115:3213–3223
3. Nieminen MS, Brutsaert D, Dickstein K, Drexler H, Follath F, Harjola VP et al (2006) EuroHeart Failure Survey II (EHFS II): a survey on hospitalized acute heart failure patients: description of population. Eur Heart J 27:2725–2736
4. Dei Cas A, Khan SS, Butler J, Mentz RJ, Bonow RO, Avogaro A et al (2015) Impact of diabetes on epidemiology, treatment, and outcomes of patients with heart failure. JACC Heart Fail 3:136–145
5. MacDonald MR, Petrie MC, Varyani F, Ostergren J, Michelson EL, Young JB et al (2008) Impact of diabetes on outcomes in patients with low and preserved ejection fraction heart failure: an analysis of the Candesartan in Heart failure: Assessment of Reduction in Mortality and morbidity (CHARM) programme. Eur Heart J 29:1377–1385
6. Owan TE, Hodge DO, Herges RM, Jacobsen SJ, Roger VL, Redfield MM (2006) Trends in prevalence and outcome of heart failure with preserved ejection fraction. N Engl J Med 355:251–259
7. Aguilar D, Deswal A, Ramasubbu K, Mann DL, Bozkurt B (2010) Comparison of patients with heart failure and preserved left ventricular ejection fraction among those with versus without diabetes mellitus. Am J Cardiol 105:373–377
8. Kapoor JR, Fonarow GC, Zhao X, Kapoor R, Hernandez AF, Heidenreich PA (2011) Diabetes, quality of care, and in-hospital outcomes in patients hospitalized with heart failure. Am Heart J 162:480–486

 9. Greenberg BH, Abraham WT, Albert NM, Chiswell K, Clare R, Stough WG et al (2007) Influence of diabetes on characteristics and outcomes in patients hospitalized with heart failure: a report from the Organized Program to Initiate Lifesaving Treatment in Hospitalized Patients with Heart Failure (OPTIMIZE-HF). Am Heart J 154:277e1–277e8

10. The SOLVD Investigators (1991) Effect of enalapril on survival in patients with reduced left ventricular ejection fractions and congestive heart failure. N Engl J Med 325:293–302

11. Ryden L, Armstrong PW, Cleland JG, Horowitz JD, Massie BM, Packer M et al (2000) Efficacy and safety of high-dose lisinopril in chronic heart failure patients at high cardiovascular risk, including those with diabetes mellitus. Results from the ATLAS trial. Eur Heart J 21:1967–1978

12. Young JB, Dunlap ME, Pfeffer MA, Probstfield JL, Cohen-Solal A, Dietz R et al (2004) Mortality and morbidity reduction with Candesartan in patients with chronic heart failure and left ventricular systolic dysfunction: results of the CHARM low-left ventricular ejection fraction trials. Circulation 110:2618–2626

13. Cohn JN, Tognoni G (2001) Valsartan Heart Failure Trial Investigators. A randomized trial of the angiotensin-receptor blocker valsartan in chronic heart failure. N Engl J Med 345:1667–1675

14. Pitt B, Remme W, Zannad F, Neaton J, Martinez F, Roniker B et al (2003) Eplerenone, a selective aldosterone blocker, in patients with left ventricular dysfunction after myocardial infarction. N Engl J Med 348:1309–1321

15. Pitt B, Zannad F, Remme WJ, Cody R, Castaigne A, Perez A et al (1999) The effect of spironolactone on morbidity and mortality in patients with severe heart failure. Randomized Aldactone Evaluation Study Investigators. N Engl J Med 341:709–717

16. Gheorghiade M, Bohm M, Greene SJ, Fonarow GC, Lewis EF, Zannad F et al (2013) Effect of aliskiren on postdischarge mortality and heart failure readmissions among patients hospitalized for heart failure: the ASTRONAUT randomized trial. JAMA 309:1125–1135

17. Yancy CW, Jessup M, Bozkurt B, Butler J, Casey DE Jr, Drazner MH et al (2013) 2013 ACCF/AHA guideline for the management of heart failure: executive summary: a report of the American College of Cardiology Foundation/American Heart Association Task Force on practice guidelines. Circulation 128:1810–1852

18. McMurray JJ, Adamopoulos S, Anker SD, Auricchio A, Bohm M, Dickstein K et al (2012) ESC Guidelines for the diagnosis and treatment of acute and chronic heart failure 2012: The Task Force for the Diagnosis and Treatment of Acute and Chronic Heart Failure 2012 of the European Society of Cardiology. Developed in collaboration with the Heart Failure Association (HFA) of the ESC. Eur Heart J 33:1787–1847

19. Minguet J, Sutton G, Ferrero C, Gomez T, Bramlage P (2015) LCZ696: a new paradigm for the treatment of heart failure? Expert Opin Pharmacother 16:435–446

20. von Lueder TG, Atar D, Krum H (2014) Current role of neprilysin inhibitors in hypertension and heart failure. Pharmacol Ther 144:41–49

21. McMurray JJ, Packer M, Desai AS, Gong J, Lefkowitz MP, Rizkala AR et al (2014) Angiotensin-neprilysin inhibition versus enalapril in heart failure. N Engl J Med 371:993–1004

22. Deedwania PC, Giles TD, Klibaner M, Ghali JK, Herlitz J, Hildebrandt P et al (2005) Efficacy, safety and tolerability of metoprolol CR/XL in patients with diabetes and chronic heart failure: experiences from MERIT-HF. Am Heart J 149:159–167

23. Erdmann E, Lechat P, Verkenne P, Wiemann H (2001) Results from post-hoc analyses of the CIBIS II trial: effect of bisoprolol in high-risk patient groups with chronic heart failure. Eur J Heart Fail 3:469–479

24. Packer M, Fowler MB, Roecker EB, Coats AJ, Katus HA, Krum H et al (2002) Effect of carvedilol on the morbidity of patients with severe chronic heart failure: results of the carvedilol prospective randomized cumulative survival (COPERNICUS) study. Circulation 106:2194–2199

25. Torp-Pedersen C, Metra M, Charlesworth A, Spark P, Lukas MA, Poole-Wilson PA et al (2007) Effects of metoprolol and carvedilol on pre-existing and new onset diabetes in patients with chronic heart failure: data from the Carvedilol Or Metoprolol European Trial (COMET). Heart 93:968–973

26. Grodin JL, Tang WH (2013) Treatment strategies for the prevention of heart failure. Curr Heart Fail Rep 10:331–340

27. Castagno D, Baird-Gunning J, Jhund PS, Biondi-Zoccai G, MacDonald MR, Petrie MC et al (2011) Intensive glycemic control has no impact on the risk of heart failure in type 2 diabetic patients: evidence from a 37,229 patient meta-analysis. Am Heart J 162:938–948

28. Erqou S, Lee CT, Adler A (2012) Intensive glycemic control and the risk of heart failure in patients with type 2 diabetes. Am Heart J 163, e35

29. Iribarren C, Karter AJ, Go AS, Ferrara A, Liu JY, Sidney S et al (2001) Glycemic control and heart failure among adult patients with diabetes. Circulation 103:2668–2673

30. Thrainsdottir IS, Aspelund T, Hardarson T, Malmberg K, Sigurdsson G, Thorgeirsson G et al (2005) Glucose abnormalities and heart failure predict poor prognosis in the population-based Reykjavik Study. Eur J Cardiovasc Prev Rehabil 12:465–471

31. Held C, Gerstein HC, Yusuf S, Zhao F, Hilbrich L, Anderson C et al (2007) Glucose levels predict hospitalization for congestive heart failure in patients at high cardiovascular risk. Circulation 115:1371–1375

Chapter 15
Ischemic Stroke

15.1 Diabetes, Atrial fibrillation, and Stroke

Ischemic stroke is a leading cause of mortality and long-term disability worldwide. Patients with DM have an increased risk of stroke and worse outcome [1–3]. This association is explained by the fact that DM people have both increased susceptibility to atherosclerosis and increased prevalence of cardiovascular (CV) risk factors such as arterial hypertension and dyslipidemia [4]. Hyperglycemia, insulin resistance, and low-grade inflammation also significantly contribute to determine a prothrombotic state characterized by increased platelet reactivity as well as disturbed coagulation cascade with increase of prothrombotic factors such as fibrinogen, thrombin, factor II, and PAI-1 [5]. The occurrence of atrial fibrillation (AF) is one of the main triggers underlying ischemic stroke in DM patients [6]. Available evidence indicates that the association between AF and DM may significantly amplify morbidity and mortality [7]. However, it remains unclear whether DM is an independent risk factor for AF. A recently published cohort study including 1,921,260 individuals, of whom 34,198 with T2D, showed a positive association of DM with ischemic stroke (1.72 [1.52–1.95]) but was not associated with

F. Paneni, F. Cosentino, *Diabetes and Cardiovascular Disease:*
A Guide to Clinical Management, DOI 10.1007/978-3-319-17762-5_15,
© Springer International Publishing Switzerland 2015

arrhythmia or sudden cardiac death (0.95 [0.76–1.19]) [8]. Along this line, the Manitoba follow-up study showed that AF was associated with DM only in univariate analysis whereas the association was lost after adjustment for covariates, indicating that other factors, namely ischemic heart disease and hypertension, may contribute to AF occurrence in diabetics [9]. By contrast, the *Framingham Heart Study* demonstrated that DM per se is associated with AF in both genders, even after adjustment for age and other risk factors (OR 1.4 for men and 1.6 for women) [10]. However, DM is not included in the Framingham risk score for AF, suggesting that other factors may better predict AF occurrence. Collectively, these data hint that the prevention of stroke in DM patients should take into account a multifactorial treatment including antihypertensive agents, statins, and glucose lowering drugs (Fig. 15.1) [11, 12]. At present, we dispose of several tools to stratify stroke risk in DM patients and this clinical information is invaluable to implement primary prevention strategies. A recent risk stratification scheme consist in the use of the CHA_2DS_2-VASc [cardiac failure, hypertension, age ≥ 75 years (doubled), DM, stroke (doubled)-vascular disease, age 65–74, and sex category (female)] [13]. This index has shown to be quite specific. Indeed, a recent study showed that patients with a CHA_2DS_2-VASc score of 0 had a truly low risk of ischemic stroke, with an annual stroke rate of approximately 1 % [14].

15.2 Pharmacological Approaches to Prevent Stroke in DM

15.2.1 Antihypertensive Treatment

Intensive control of blood pressure (BP) significantly reduces stroke risk in DM patients. In the UKPDS study, mean BP during follow up was significantly reduced in the group assigned to

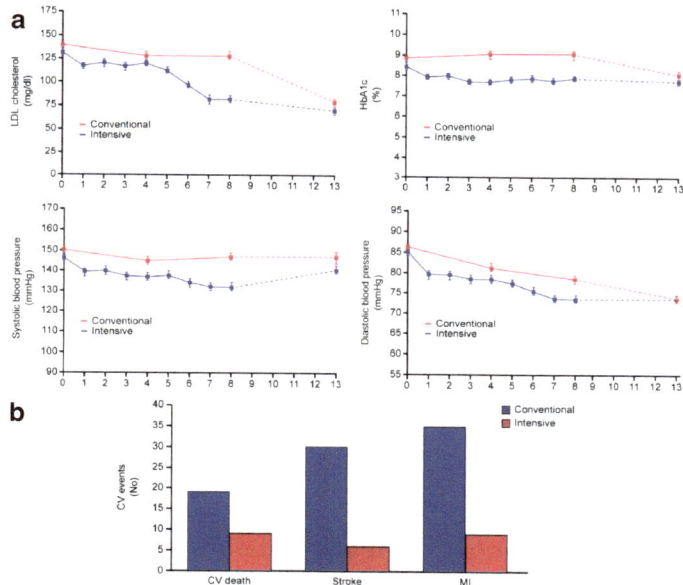

Fig. 15.1 (**a**) Multifactorial control of cardiovascular risk factors and (**b**) occurrence of cardiovascular outcomes, including stroke (Data from Gaede et al. [12])

tight BP control (144/82 mmHg) compared with the group assigned to less tight control (154/87 mmHg) ($p < 0.0001$) [15]. Such BP reduction was associated with a 44 % decrease in the risk of stroke (CI 11–65, $p = 0.013$). Other studies have shown that even small BP reduction may be sufficient to reduce stroke risk. In the HOPE study, BP reduction with ramipril was modest (3.8 mmHg systolic and 2.8 mmHg diastolic) but the relative risk of any stroke was reduced by 32 % as compared to placebo whereas risk of fatal stroke decreased by 61 %. This study did not clarify whether these benefits represent a specific effect of ACE inhibitors or were simply the result of BP lowering [16].

The more recent ADVANCE and ACCORD trials did not confirm the benefits of intensive BP reduction on stroke risk in DM patients [17, 18]. A recent meta-analysis showed that intensive BP control was associated with a 17 % reduction in stroke, and a 20 % increase in serious adverse effects as compared with standard BP control [19]. More intensive BP control ($\leq$130 mmHg) was associated with a greater reduction in stroke, but did not reduce other events. Based on these evidence, current recommendation suggest that people with DM and hypertension should be treated to a systolic blood pressure (SBP) goal of <40 mmHg and a DBP <85 mmHg [11, 13, 20].

15.2.2   Lipid-Lowering Therapies

Reduction of LDL cholesterol levels reduces the risk of stroke in DM patients whereas the available evidence does not support a benefit from drugs targeting triglycerides and HDL cholesterol. In the CARDS trial (*Collaborative Atorvastatin Diabetes Study*) treatment with atorvastatin 10 mg in 2,800 patients with T2D decreased the risk of stroke by 48 % [21]. In a meta-analysis of 14 randomized controlled trials including more than 18,000 persons with DM, the mean duration of follow-up was 4.3 years, with 3,247 major vascular events. The study reported a 9 % reduction in all-cause mortality and a significant reduction in stroke risk (0.79, 0.67–0.93; $p = 0.0002$) [22]. Interestingly, these effects were proportional to the mmol/L reduction in LDL cholesterol. In contrast, fibrate therapy is not associated with a significant reduction on the risk of stroke (RR, 1.02, 95 % CI, 0.90–1.16, $p = 0.78$), as reported in a recent meta-analysis including 37,791 patients [23]. However, a subgroup analysis showed that fibrate therapy may reduce fatal stroke (RR, 0.49, 95 % CI, 0.26–0.93, $p = 0.03$) in patients with previous DM or CVD [23]. The benefit of HDL raising therapies on stroke risk is also inconclusive and not supported by evidence. Treatment with niacin in the AIM-HIGH trial (Atherothrombosis Intervention in Metabolic Syndrome with Low HDL/High Triglycerides) was effective in modulating TG and HDL levels but not in reducing stroke [24]. Along the same line, treatment with the CETP inhibitors torcetrapib and dalcetrapib did not reduce the rates of fatal and nonfatal stroke despite a consistent increase of HDL levels [25].

15.2.3   Antidiabetic Medications

The recent randomized trial ACCORD, ADVANCE, and VADT were unable to show that intensive glycemic control targeting HbA1c <6.5 % or <6 % reduces the risk of stroke in DM patients [26]. Hence, from these results there is no evidence that reduced glycemia decreases the mid-term risk of macrovascular events including stroke [11]. Current recommendation suggest that HbA_{1c} should be reduced <7 % to prevent microvascular complications, yet it remains unclear whether control to this level may also reduce the risk of stroke [27]. A recent meta-analysis of 9 randomized trials including 59,197 patients showed that, overall, intensive control of glucose as compared to standard care had no effect on incident stroke (RR, 0.96; 95 %CI 0.88–1.06; $p=0.445$) [28]. However, in the stratified analyses, a beneficial effect was seen in those patients having body mass index (BMI)>30 (RR, 0.86; 95 %CI: 0.75–0.99; $p=0.041$), suggesting a potential benefit among obese individuals [28]. Despite the lack of convincing support from large trials, there is evidence that some glucose-lowering drugs may affect stroke risk. A recent study demonstrated that patients who were on sulfonylureas prior to stroke and continued to receive these agents during hospitalization were more likely to have a better neurological and functional outcome at discharge [29]. However, a meta-analysis including 33 studies ($n=1,325,446$ patients) reported that sulphonylureas use was associated with a significantly increased risk of CV events, including stroke [30]. In studies comparing sulphonylureas vs. metformin, these relative risks were 1.26 (95 % CI 1.17–1.35) and 1.18 (95 % CI 1.13–1.24), respectively [30]. Treatment with metformin was associated with a decreased risk of CV mortality (pooled OR, 0.74; 95 % CI, 0.62–0.89) compared with any other oral glucose-lowering agent or placebo; however, the results for CV morbidity, stroke, and all-cause mortality were similar but not statistically significant [31]. A meta-analysis including 94 trials enrolling 85,224 patients (median follow-up 29 weeks) showed that treatment with DPP-4 inhibitors did not affect all-cause and CV mortality, as well as stroke, in the short and long terms (<29 weeks and >29 weeks, respectively) [32]. Recent evidence suggests that GLP-1 receptor agonists were associated with a significant reduction in the incidence of major CV events (including stroke) as compared with placebo and pioglitazone [33].

15.3   Stroke Prevention in Diabetic Patients With Atrial Fibrillation

15.3.1   Warfarin

Warfarin has generally been the treatment of choice for patients at high risk for cardioembolic stroke and low risk of hemorrhagic complications [34]. This benefit is outlined by primary and secondary prevention studies including 2,900 patients with an overall 62 % reduction of relative risk (95 % CI 48–72). Warfarin is more effective than aspirin alone [RR 39 % (95 % CI, 22–25)] or aspirin plus clopidrogrel [RR 60 % (95 % CI 18–56), both in patients with and without DM [11]. However, oral anticoagulation with warfarin increases major extracranial bleedings by 0.3 % per year [13].

15.3.2   Dabigatran

In the *Randomized Evaluation of Long-Term Anticoagulant Therapy* (RE-LY) study, the direct thrombin inhibitor dabigatran given at a dose of 110 mg was associated with rates of stroke and systemic embolism that were similar to those associated with warfarin, as well as lower rates of major hemorrhage [35]. Moreover, dabigatran administered at a dose of 150 mg, as compared to warfarin, was associated with lower rates of stroke and systemic embolism but similar rates of major hemorrhage (Table 15.1). Of note, the benefits of dabigatran were more pronounced among DM patients, although this difference did not achieve significance due to low statistical power [35].

15.3.3   Apixaban

The factor Xa inhibitor apixaban, administered at the dose of 5 mg b.i.d. demonstrated a significant benefit when compared to aspirin (81–324 mg) in the *The Apixaban VERsus acetylsalicylic acid to pRevent strOkES* (AVERROES) trial [36]. More recently, the *Apixaban for Reduction in Stroke and Other Thromboembolic Events in Atrial Fibrillation* (ARISTOTLE) trial showed that in patients with AF, apixaban was superior to warfarin in preventing stroke or systemic embolism (0.66–0.95; $p < 0.001$ for noninferiority; $p = 0.01$ for superiority), caused less bleeding, and resulted in lower mortality [37]. Apixaban-related benefits were also observed in the subgroup of 4,547 DM patients with 1.4 events as compared to 1.9 % observed with warfarin. However, significance was reached only among non-DM subjects ($n = 13,654$) [37].

Table 15.1 Major trials comparing new anticoagulants with aspirin and warfarin in patients with atrial fibrillation at risk for stroke

Trial	Population	Intervention	Stroke risk	Bleeding risk	Implications
RE-LY	18,113 patients with AF at risk for stroke	Fixed doses of dabigatran (110 mg or 150 mg twice daily) vs. adjusted-dose warfarin	Dabigatran 110 mg (RR, 0.91; 95 % CI, 0.74–1.11; $p<0.001$, for noninferiority) Dabigatran 150 mg (RR, 0.66; 95 % CI, 0.53–0.82; $p<0.001$, for superiority)	Dabigatran 110 mg vs. warfarin (2.71 % vs. 3.36 % per year, $p=0.003$) Dabigatran 150 mg vs. warfarin (2.71 % vs. 3.11 % per year, $p=0.31$)	Dabigatran 110 mg was associated with rates of stroke and systemic embolism similar to warfarin, but lower rates of major hemorrhage Dabigatran 150 mg was associated with lower rates of stroke and systemic embolism as compared to warfarin, but similar rates of major hemorrhage

AVERROES	5,599 patients with AF at risk for stroke, for whom VKAs were unsuitable	Apixaban (5 mg twice daily) vs. Aspirin (81–324 mg daily)	The study was stopped early because of a clear benefit of apixaban in reducing stroke and systemic embolism (HR with apixaban, 0.45; 95 % CI, 0.32–0.62; $p < 0.001$) as well as death (HR, 0.79; 95 % CI, 0.62–1.02; $p = 0.07$).	Aspirin vs. apixaban (HR, 1.13; 95 % CI, 0.74–1.75; $p = 0.57$)	In AF patients for whom VKAs therapy is unsuitable, apixaban reduced the risk of stroke or systemic embolism without significantly increasing the risk of major bleeding or intracranial hemorrhage
ARISTOTLE	18,201 patients with AF and at least one additional risk factor for stroke	Apixaban (5 mg twice daily) vs. adjusted-dose warfarin	Compared to warfarin, apixaban significantly reduced ischemic stroke and systemic embolism (HR 0.79; 95 % CI, 0.66–0.95; $p < 0.001$ for noninferiority; $p = 0.01$ for superiority)	Apixaban vs. warfarin (HR, 0.69; 95 % CI, 0.60–0.80; $p < 0.001$)	In AF patients, apixaban was superior to warfarin in preventing stroke or systemic embolism, caused less bleeding, and resulted in lower mortality

(continued)

Table 15.1 (continued)

Trial	Population	Intervention	Stroke risk	Bleeding risk	Implications
ROCKET	14,264 AF patients at increased risk for stroke	Rivaroxaban (20 mg daily) vs. dose-adjusted warfarin	Compared to warfarin, rivaroxaban significantly reduced ischemic stroke and systemic embolism (HR, 0.79; 95 % CI, 0.66–0.96; $p < 0.001$ for noninferiority)	Rivaroxaban vs. warfarin (HR, 1.03; 95 % CI, 0.96–1.11; $p = 0.44$) Rivaroxaban significantly reduced intracranial hemorrhage (0.5 % vs. 0.7 %, $p = 0.02$) and fatal bleeding (0.2 % vs. 0.5 %, $p = 0.003$)	In AF patients, rivaroxaban was noninferior to warfarin for the prevention of stroke or systemic embolism There was no significant between-group difference in the risk of major bleeding, although intracranial and fatal bleeding occurred less frequently in the rivaroxaban group.

AF atrial fibrillation, *VKAs* vitamin K antagonists, *HR* hazard ratio

15.3.4   *Rivaroxaban*

The *Rivaroxaban Once Daily Oral Direct Factor Xa Inhibition Compared with Vitamin K Antagonism for Prevention of Stroke and Embolism Trial in Atrial Fibrillation* (ROCKET) trial, comparing warfarin with rivaroxaban, showed the noninferiority of rivaroxaban to warfarin in preventing stroke, systemic embolism, or major bleeding among the AF patients with a relatively high $CHADS_2$ score (median 3.5) [38]. In conclusion, these new oral anticoagulants have the potential to be used as an alternative to warfarin, especially in patients intolerant to – or unsuitable for – vitamin K antagonists. In analyses of prespecified subgroups in the ROCKET trial, patients with DM had a level of protection similar to the overall study populations (Table 15.1) [11, 39].

References

1. Arboix A (2009) Stroke prognosis in diabetes mellitus: new insights but questions remain. Expert Rev Cardiovasc Ther 7:1181–1185
2. Mankovsky BN, Ziegler D (2004) Stroke in patients with diabetes mellitus. Diabetes Metab Res Rev 20:268–287
3. Banerjee C, Moon YP, Paik MC, Rundek T, Mora-McLaughlin C, Vieira JR et al (2012) Duration of diabetes and risk of ischemic stroke: the Northern Manhattan Study. Stroke 43:1212–1217
4. Benson RT, Sacco RL (2000) Stroke prevention: hypertension, diabetes, tobacco, and lipids. Neurol Clin 18:309–319
5. Paneni F, Beckman JA, Creager MA, Cosentino F (2013) Diabetes and vascular disease: pathophysiology, clinical consequences, and medical therapy: part I. Eur Heart J 34:2436–2443
6. McFarlane SI, Sica DA, Sowers JR (2005) Stroke in patients with diabetes and hypertension. J Clin Hypertens 7:286–292
7. Boden-Albala B, Cammack S, Chong J, Wang C, Wright C, Rundek T et al (2008) Diabetes, fasting glucose levels, and risk of ischemic stroke and vascular events: findings from the Northern Manhattan Study (NOMAS). Diabetes Care 31:1132–1137

8. Shah AD, Langenberg C, Rapsomaniki E, Denaxas S, Pujades-Rodriguez M, Gale CP et al (2015) Type 2 diabetes and incidence of cardiovascular diseases: a cohort study in 1.9 million people. Lancet Diabetes Endocrinol 3:105–113

9. Krahn AD, Manfreda J, Tate RB, Mathewson FA, Cuddy TE (1995) The natural history of atrial fibrillation: incidence, risk factors, and prognosis in the Manitoba Follow-Up Study. Am J Med 98:476–484

10. Benjamin EJ, Levy D, Vaziri SM, D'Agostino RB, Belanger AJ, Wolf PA (1994) Independent risk factors for atrial fibrillation in a population-based cohort. The Framingham Heart Study. JAMA 271:840–844

11. Meschia JF, Bushnell C, Boden-Albala B, Braun LT, Bravata DM, Chaturvedi S et al (2014) Guidelines for the primary prevention of stroke: a statement for healthcare professionals from the American Heart Association/American Stroke Association. Stroke 45: 3754–3832

12. Gaede P, Lund-Andersen H, Parving HH, Pedersen O (2008) Effect of a multifactorial intervention on mortality in type 2 diabetes. N Engl J Med 358:580–591

13. Ryden L, Grant PJ, Anker SD, Berne C, Cosentino F, Danchin N et al (2013) ESC Guidelines on diabetes, pre-diabetes, and cardiovascular diseases developed in collaboration with the EASD: the Task Force on diabetes, pre-diabetes, and cardiovascular diseases of the European Society of Cardiology (ESC) and developed in collaboration with the European Association for the Study of Diabetes (EASD). Eur Heart J 34:3035–3087

14. Chao TF, Liu CJ, Wang KL, Lin YJ, Chang SL, Lo LW et al (2014) Using the CHA2DS2-VASc score for refining stroke risk stratification in "low-risk" Asian patients with atrial fibrillation. J Am Coll Cardiol 64:1658–1665

15. Holman RR, Paul SK, Bethel MA, Matthews DR, Neil HA (2008) 10-year follow-up of intensive glucose control in type 2 diabetes. N Engl J Med 359:1577–1589

16. Heart Outcomes Prevention Evaluation Study Investigators (2000) Effects of ramipril on cardiovascular and microvascular outcomes in people with diabetes mellitus: results of the HOPE study and MICRO-HOPE substudy. Lancet 355:253–259

17. Gerstein HC, Miller ME, Byington RP, Goff DC Jr, Bigger JT, Buse JB et al (2008) Effects of intensive glucose lowering in type 2 diabetes. N Engl J Med 358:2545–2559

18. Patel A, MacMahon S, Chalmers J, Neal B, Billot L, Woodward M et al (2008) Intensive blood glucose control and vascular outcomes in patients with type 2 diabetes. N Engl J Med 358:2560–2572

19. Bangalore S, Kumar S, Lobach I, Messerli FH (2011) Blood pressure targets in subjects with type 2 diabetes mellitus/impaired fasting glucose: observations from traditional and bayesian random-effects meta-analyses of randomized trials. Circulation 123:2799–2810

20. Mancia G, Fagard R, Narkiewicz K, Redon J, Zanchetti A, Bohm M et al (2013) 2013 ESH/ESC guidelines for the management of arterial hypertension: the Task Force for the Management of Arterial Hypertension of the European Society of Hypertension (ESH) and of the European Society of Cardiology (ESC). Eur Heart J 34:2159–2219

21. Colhoun HM, Betteridge DJ, Durrington PN, Hitman GA, Neil HA, Livingstone SJ et al (2004) Primary prevention of cardiovascular disease with atorvastatin in type 2 diabetes in the Collaborative Atorvastatin Diabetes Study (CARDS): multicentre randomised placebo-controlled trial. Lancet 364:685–696

22. Kearney PM, Blackwell L, Collins R, Keech A, Simes J, Peto R et al (2008) Efficacy of cholesterol-lowering therapy in 18,686 people with diabetes in 14 randomised trials of statins: a meta-analysis. Lancet 371:117–125

23. Amarenco P, Labreuche J (2009) Lipid management in the prevention of stroke: review and updated meta-analysis of statins for stroke prevention. Lancet Neurol 8:453–463

24. Boden WE, Probstfield JL, Anderson T, Chaitman BR, Desvignes-Nickens P, Koprowicz K et al (2011) Niacin in patients with low HDL cholesterol levels receiving intensive statin therapy. N Engl J Med 365: 2255–2267

25. Landmesser U, von Eckardstein A, Kastelein J, Deanfield J, Luscher TF (2012) Increasing high-density lipoprotein cholesterol by cholesteryl ester transfer protein-inhibition: a rocky road and lessons learned? The early demise of the dal-HEART programme. Eur Heart J 33:1712–1715

26. Skyler JS, Bergenstal R, Bonow RO, Buse J, Deedwania P, Gale EA et al (2009) Intensive glycemic control and the prevention of cardiovascular events: implications of the ACCORD, ADVANCE, and VA Diabetes Trials: a position statement of the American Diabetes Association and a Scientific Statement of the American College of Cardiology Foundation and the American Heart Association. J Am Coll Cardiol 53:298–304

27. American Diabetes Association (2014) Standards of medical care in diabetes – 2014. Diabetes Care 37(Suppl 1):S14–S80

28. Zhang C, Zhou YH, Xu CL, Chi FL, Ju HN (2013) Efficacy of intensive control of glucose in stroke prevention: a meta-analysis of data from 59,197 participants in 9 randomized controlled trials. PLoS One 8, e54465

29. Kunte H, Schmidt S, Eliasziw M, del Zoppo GJ, Simard JM, Masuhr F et al (2007) Sulfonylureas improve outcome in patients with type 2 diabetes and acute ischemic stroke. Stroke 38:2526–2530

30. Phung OJ, Schwartzman E, Allen RW, Engel SS, Rajpathak SN (2013) Sulphonylureas and risk of cardiovascular disease: systematic review and meta-analysis. Diabet Med 30:1160–1171

31. Magkou D, Tziomalos K (2014) Antidiabetic treatment, stroke severity and outcome. World J Diabetes 5:84–88

32. Savarese G, Perrone-Filardi P, D'Amore C, Vitale C, Trimarco B, Pani L et al (2014) Cardiovascular effects of dipeptidyl peptidase-4 inhibitors in diabetic patients: A meta-analysis. Int J Cardiol 181C:239–244

33. Monami M, Dicembrini I, Nardini C, Fiordelli I, Mannucci E (2014) Effects of glucagon-like peptide-1 receptor agonists on cardiovascular risk: a meta-analysis of randomized clinical trials. Diabetes Obes Metab 16:38–47

34. Blackshear JL, Kusumoto F (2005) Stroke prevention in atrial fibrillation: warfarin faces its challengers. Curr Cardiol Rep 7:16–22

35. Connolly SJ, Ezekowitz MD, Yusuf S, Eikelboom J, Oldgren J, Parekh A et al (2009) Dabigatran versus warfarin in patients with atrial fibrillation. N Engl J Med 361:1139–1151

36. Connolly SJ, Eikelboom J, Joyner C, Diener HC, Hart R, Golitsyn S et al (2011) Apixaban in patients with atrial fibrillation. N Engl J Med 364:806–817

37. Granger CB, Alexander JH, McMurray JJ, Lopes RD, Hylek EM, Hanna M et al (2011) Apixaban versus warfarin in patients with atrial fibrillation. N Engl J Med 365:981–992

38. Patel MR, Mahaffey KW, Garg J, Pan G, Singer DE, Hacke W et al (2011) Rivaroxaban versus warfarin in nonvalvular atrial fibrillation. N Engl J Med 365:883–891

39. Lega JC, Bertoletti L, Gremillet C, Chapelle C, Mismetti P, Cucherat M et al (2014) Consistency of safety and efficacy of new oral anticoagulants across subgroups of patients with atrial fibrillation. PLoS One 9, e91398

Chapter 16
Peripheral Artery Disease

16.1   Prevalence and Prognosis

Diabetes mellitus (DM) is associated with accelerated athero-sclerosis occurring at different arterial districts including carotid arteries, aorta, femoral arteries, and lower extremities [1]. A recent cohort study including almost two million individuals showed that peripheral artery disease (PAD) is the most common complication observed among T2D people with a first cardiovascular presentation, being reported in 992 (16.2 %) of 6,137 patients [2]. Of note, PAD in DM patients was the most prevalent disorder as compared to heart failure, stroke, stable angina, and myocardial infarction (Fig. 16.1) [2]. Furthermore, of 12 cardiovascular disease studied, PAD showed the strongest association with T2D, with an adjusted HR of 2.98 (95 % CI 2.76–3.22) (Table 16.1) [2]. This observation is in line with the notion that the incidence of MI and stroke has declined rapidly during the past few decades [3]. Global estimates report that prevalence of PAD at age 45–49 years is 5.28 % in women and 5.41 % in men, while reaching 18.38 % in women and 18.83 % in men at the age 85–89 years [4]. A Health Professionals Follow-up Study conducted in DM men demonstrated that duration of DM is a potent predictor of incident PAD (Table 16.2)

F. Paneni, F. Cosentino, *Diabetes and Cardiovascular Disease:* 203
A Guide to Clinical Management, DOI 10.1007/978-3-319-17762-5_16,
© Springer International Publishing Switzerland 2015

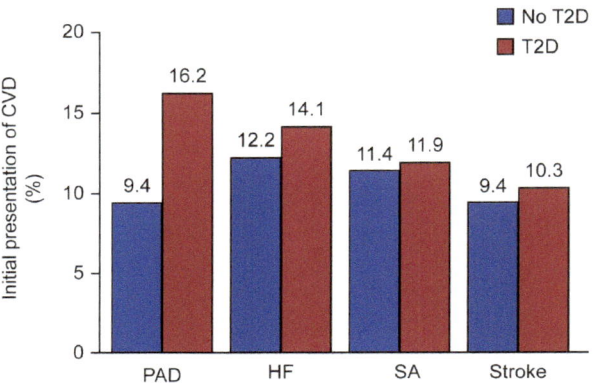

Fig. 16.1 Distribution of initial presentations of cardiovascular disease in participants with and without type 2 diabetes and no history of cardiovascular disease (Data from Shah et al. [2])

Table 16.1 Adjusted hazard ratios (HRs) for different initial presentations of cardiovascular diseases associated with type 2 diabetes, adjusted for age, sex, BMI, deprivation, HDL cholesterol, total cholesterol, systolic blood pressure, smoking status, statin, and antihypertensive drug prescriptions

Presentation of CVD	Number of events		HR (95 % CI)	p value
	No T2D	T2D		
Stable angina	12,232	728	1.62 (1.49–1.77)	<0.0001
Nonfatal myocardial infarction	15,191	706	1.54 (1.42–1.67)	<0.0001
Heart failure	15,072	866	1.56 (1.45–1.69)	<0.0001
Arrhythmia or sudden cardiac death	3,218	100	0.95 (0.76–1.19)	0.65
Ischemic stroke	5,643	316	1.72 (1.52–1.95)	<0.0001
Peripheral arterial disease	10,076	992	2.98 (2.76–3.22)	<0.0001

Data from Shah et al. [2]

Table 16.2 Multivariate adjusted relative risk of peripheral artery disease according to diabetes duration

Duration of diabetes (years)	Relative risk of PAD (95 % confidence interval)
1–5	1.39 (0.82–2.36)
6–10	3.63 (2.23–5.88)
11–25	2.55 (1.50–4.32)
>25	4.53 (2.39–8.58)

Data from Al-Delaimy et al. [5]

[5]. Moreover, poor glycemic control is an independent risk factor for PAD. Indeed, every 1 % increase in glycosylated hemoglobin (HbA_{1c}) increases PAD risk by 28 % [6]. Patients with DM also tend to present with multisite atherosclerosis as compared to non-DM, and this affects prognosis [7, 8]. The location of the disease has been associated with different outcomes. Older age, male sex, DM, heart failure, and critical limb ischemia are associated with distal disease, whereas female sex, smoking, hypertension, dyslipidemia, coronary heart disease, cerebrovascular disease, and chronic obstructive pulmonary disease are usually associated with proximal disease [9]. However, proximal disease does not seem to be associated with mortality, whereas the association of distal disease with death remains significant even after correction for relevant confounders (HR, 1.2; 95 % CI, 1.1–1.3) [9].

16.2 Diagnosis

Most of atherosclerotic lesions in DM patients are observed in the popliteal artery or in vessels of the lower leg [10]. Typical presentation of PAD includes intermittent claudication, fatigue, arching, cramping, and rest pain, with the location of symptoms relating to the site of proximal stenosis [11]. For the clinical diagnosis, the palpation of pulses and visual inspections of feet are an essential step. Unfortunately, the majority (90 %) of DM do not have symptoms and diagnosis is made at an advanced stage of the disease. In a prospective cohort study including 6,880 patients aged ≥65 years, 5,392 patients had no PAD, 836 had asymptomatic PAD (ankle brachial index <0.9 without symptoms), and 593 had symptomatic PAD [12]. Of note, the risk of mortality was similar in symptomatic and asymptomatic patients with PAD and was significantly higher than in those without PAD, suggesting the importance of diagnosing PAD.

PAD can be classified into five stages, according to the classification proposed by Fontaine: stage I (asymptomatic), stage IIa (mild claudication), stage IIb (moderate to severe claudication), stage III (rest pain), and stage IV (ulceration or gangrene) [13]. The early detection of atherosclerosis in patients with DM is instrumental for reclassification into different risk categories, requiring aggressive therapeutic regimens. Therefore, reliable indicators of PAD are in high demand for the primary prevention of CVD in DM. A reliable indicator of PAD is the ankle brachial index (ABI) (Table 16.3) [14]. This test is done by measuring blood pressure at the ankle (posterior tibial or dorsalis pedal level) and in the arm (brachial systolic blood pressure) while a person is at rest. Several noninvasive techniques are used to detect limb flow or pulse volume for measuring the ABI, primarily Doppler ultrasound and oscillometric methods. The former uses a continuous-wave Doppler probe for the detection of arterial flow [14]. The overall diagnostic ability is higher for ABI measured by Doppler than that measured with the oscillometric method [15, 16]. However, lower sensitivities have been reported in DM patients [14]. An ABI <0.9 indicates PAD with high probability, whereas an ABI <0.8 is sufficient to diagnose PAD, regardless of symptoms. Lower ABI values indicate more severe PAD (Table 16.3) [17]. Patients with symptoms or claudication generally have ABI from 0.5 to 0.8, while in patients with critical limb ischemia ABI is usually below 0.5. In 6,986

Table 16.3 ABI values, clinical presentation, and treatment options for peripheral artery disease in patients with diabetes

ABI	Relative risk of PAD (95 % CI)	Clinical presentation	Recommendation
1–1.40	Normal	Asymptomatic	Annual visits to measure ABI
0.90–1	Borderline value suggestive of increased CV risk, regardless of PAD symptoms and other CV risk factors	Asymptomatic	Postexercise ABI or other noninvasive tests, which may include imaging, should be used
0.80–0.90	Very high probability of PAD	Asymptomatic or mild claudication	If uncertainties remain, postexercise ABI or other noninvasive tests, which may include imaging, should be used. Supervised exercise programs, intensive multifactorial management, and cilostazol/pentoxifyilline are encouraged

(continued)

Table 16.3 (continued)

ABI	Relative risk of PAD (95 % CI)	Clinical presentation	Recommendation
0.5–0.8	Severe PAD, claudicatio intermittens	Moderate to severe claudication or rest pain	Supervised exercise programs, intensive multifactorial management, cilostazol/ pentoxifylline to control symptoms Perform angiography for further anatomic definition if lifestyle limiting symptoms persist or there is evidence of inflow disease Consider endovascular therapy or surgical bypass
<0.4	Advanced PAD, less than 40 % can complete the 6-min walking test	Severe claudication Rest pain Ulceration or gangrene	Multifactorial management Consider endovascular therapy or surgical bypass
>1.40	Consider PAD. This value suggests increased CV risk, regardless of PAD symptoms and other CV risk factors	Asymptomatic	Toe-brachial index or other noninvasive tests, which may include imaging, should be used

ABI ankle brachial index, *PAD* peripheral artery disease, *CV* cardiovascular

participants from the REACH registry, a low ABI was associated with CV mortality (HR, 1.98, 95 % CI 1.62–2.41) and all-cause mortality (HR 2.01, 95 % CI 1.72–2.36) [18]. An ABI > 1.4 indicates arterial stiffness and reduced vessel compliance as the result of medial calcinosis (Table 16.3) [19, 20]. The latter is frequently observed in DM patients and predicts prognosis. Indeed, high ABI values are associated with higher risk of all-cause mortality in DM individuals (HR 2.11, 95 % CI 1.16–3.84), but not in persons without DM (HR 0.82, 95 % CI 0.36–1.85) [18]. ABI can also be assessed by an exercise test. In this case, blood pressure measurements are repeated at both sites after a few minutes of walking on a treadmill [14]. Postexercise ABI may identify significant PAD even in people with a normal resting ABI [21]. Current recommendations from the American Diabetes Association (ADA) suggest that a screening ABI should be performed in all DM patients > 50 years or in anyone with symptoms consistent with PAD [22].

16.3 Pharmacological and Nonpharmacological Treatment

The firs aim in DM patients with PAD is to aggressively intervene on modifiable CV risk factors to combat atherosclerotic burden [19]. Smoking cessation is significantly associated with reduced risk of PAD. However, recent evidence suggest that an increased occurrence of PAD persists even among former smokers who maintain abstinence [23]. Physical exercise may also improve quality of life and symptoms in PAD patients [24]. Recent evidence indicates that supervised exercise therapy is able to ameliorate physical activity and ambulatory activities in patients with intermittent claudication [25, 26]. A meta-analysis including both randomized and not randomized trials showed that pain-free walking time was improved by

179 % and maximal walking time was improved by 122 % in patients with claudication who underwent supervised exercise training [27]. In PAD patients, a combination therapy including drugs and exercise is often used. In the Steno-2 Study, where 160 T2D patients with persistent microalbuminuria were assigned to receive either intensive or conventional therapy, the risk of amputation was significantly reduced in the intensive arm (10 vs. 33 events) [28]. Several studies suggest that statins may improve clinical features of PAD in DM patients. Simvastatin treatment was associated with improved walking distance and pain-free survival [29]. Similarly, patients receiving atorvastatin had an increased pain-free walking distance and less annual decline in lower-extremity performance [30]. The ABCD trial showed that intensive blood pressure reduction to a mean of 128/75 mmHg resulted in marked decrease of CV morbidity and mortality in PAD patients with an ABI <0.9 [31]. However, other studies with beta-blockers or alpha adrenergic blockers have shown that significant reductions in systolic BP significantly worsened walking distance. Therefore, BP reduction should not be too strong in these patients, in accordance with current guidelines [32]. The benefits of aspirin remain highly debated in DM patients with PAD. The *Aspirin for Asymptomatic Atherosclerosis* trial performed in patients aged 50–70 with an ABI value <0.95 failed to show a benefit of aspirin after 8.2 years follow-up [33]. Moreover, a meta-analysis including 5,269 patients with PAD showed that treatment with aspirin alone resulted in a statistically nonsignificant decrease in the primary end point of CV events and a significant reduction in nonfatal stroke [34]. By contrast, data from the Antithrombotic Trialists' Collaboration demonstrated that aspirin reduced CV events in the subgroup of 9,000 patients with PAD [35]. Based on available evidence, current guidelines recommend aspirin for symptomatic patients (class I) and asymptomatic patients with PAD (class II) [19]. Cilostazol, naftidrofuryl, and pentoxifylline increase walking distance in

patients with intermittent claudication, but their role remains uncertain. A recent pooled analysis showed that cilostazol improves walking distance in people with intermittent claudication secondary to PAD despite this treatment being associated with mild adverse side effects, which are generally treatable [36]. At present, there is insufficient data on whether taking cilostazol results in a reduction of all-cause mortality and cardiovascular events or an improvement in quality of life. Future research into the effect of cilostazol on intermittent claudication is warranted [19].

16.4 Endovascular and Surgical Management

A large proportion of patients with PAD complain symptoms despite maximal medical therapy and exercise programs. In these patients, further imaging is required to better define vascular anatomy before proceeding with revascularization strategies [19]. Two general approaches are being used in PAD patients: endovascular interventions and open surgical techniques. Medicare claims data from 1996 to 2006 reveal an almost doubling of lower extremity vascular procedures: the use of endovascular repair increased more than threefold, bypass surgery decreased 42 %, and the amputation rate decreased by 29 % [37]. Percutaneous approach is generally the treatment of choice in patients with focal lesions in arteries above the knee, with the best results observed for aortoiliac vessels [19, 38]. Surgical revascularization is indicated in patients with acceptable surgical risk who require a more durable repair, in those with lesions technically unsuitable for endovascular repair, and in patients who experienced failure of endovascular repair. Surgery remains the best approach in DM patients with chronic limb ischemia with the aim of healing ulcers and preventing limb loss [38].

References

1. Jude EB, Eleftheriadou I, Tentolouris N (2010) Peripheral arterial disease in diabetes – a review. Diabet Med 27:4–14
2. Shah AD, Langenberg C, Rapsomaniki E, Denaxas S, Pujades-Rodriguez M, Gale CP et al (2015) Type 2 diabetes and incidence of cardiovascular diseases: a cohort study in 1.9 million people. Lancet Diabetes Endocrinol 3:105–113
3. van Dieren S, Beulens JW, van der Schouw YT, Grobbee DE, Neal B (2010) The global burden of diabetes and its complications: an emerging pandemic. Eur J Cardiovasc Prev Rehabil 17(Suppl 1):S3–S8
4. Fowkes FG, Rudan D, Rudan I, Aboyans V, Denenberg JO, McDermott MM et al (2013) Comparison of global estimates of prevalence and risk factors for peripheral artery disease in 2000 and 2010: a systematic review and analysis. Lancet 382:1329–1340
5. Al-Delaimy WK, Merchant AT, Rimm EB, Willett WC, Stampfer MJ, Hu FB (2004) Effect of type 2 diabetes and its duration on the risk of peripheral arterial disease among men. Am J Med 116:236–240
6. Selvin E, Marinopoulos S, Berkenblit G, Rami T, Brancati FL, Powe NR et al (2004) Meta-analysis: glycosylated hemoglobin and cardiovascular disease in diabetes mellitus. Ann Intern Med 141:421–431
7. Ferrieres J, Cambou JP, Gayet JL, Herrmann MA, Leizorovicz A (2006) Prognosis of patients with atherothrombotic disease: a prospective survey in a non-hospital setting. Int J Cardiol 112:302–307
8. Alberts MJ, Bhatt DL, Mas JL, Ohman EM, Hirsch AT, Rother J et al (2009) Three-year follow-up and event rates in the international REduction of Atherothrombosis for Continued Health Registry. Eur Heart J 30:2318–2326
9. Chen Q, Smith CY, Bailey KR, Wennberg PW, Kullo IJ (2013) Disease location is associated with survival in patients with peripheral arterial disease. J Am Heart Assoc 2:e000304
10. Dinh T, Scovell S, Veves A (2009) Peripheral arterial disease and diabetes: a clinical update. Int J Low Extrem Wounds 8:75–81
11. Hittel N, Donnelly R (2002) Treating peripheral arterial disease in patients with diabetes. Diabetes Obes Metab 4(Suppl 2):S26–S31
12. Diehm C, Allenberg JR, Pittrow D, Mahn M, Tepohl G, Haberl RL et al (2009) Mortality and vascular morbidity in older adults with asymptomatic versus symptomatic peripheral artery disease. Circulation 120:2053–2061
13. White CJ, Gray WA (2007) Endovascular therapies for peripheral arterial disease: an evidence-based review. Circulation 116:2203–2215

14. Aboyans V, Criqui MH, Abraham P, Allison MA, Creager MA, Diehm C et al (2012) Measurement and interpretation of the ankle-brachial index: a scientific statement from the American Heart Association. Circulation 126:2890–2909

15. Clairotte C, Retout S, Potier L, Roussel R, Escoubet B (2009) Automated ankle-brachial pressure index measurement by clinical staff for peripheral arterial disease diagnosis in nondiabetic and diabetic patients. Diabetes Care 32:1231–1236

16. Guo X, Li J, Pang W, Zhao M, Luo Y, Sun Y et al (2008) Sensitivity and specificity of ankle-brachial index for detecting angiographic stenosis of peripheral arteries. Circ J 72:605–610

17. Ali Z, Ahmed SM, Bhutto AR, Chaudhry A, Munir SM (2012) Peripheral artery disease in type II diabetes. J Coll Physicians Surg Pak 22:686–689

18. Potier L, Roussel R, Labreuche J, Marre M, Cacoub P, Rother J et al (2014) Interaction between diabetes and a high ankle-brachial index on mortality risk. Eur J Prev Cardiol. doi:10.1177/2047487314533621

19. Rooke TW, Hirsch AT, Misra S, Sidawy AN, Beckman JA, Findeiss L et al (2013) Management of patients with peripheral artery disease (compilation of 2005 and 2011 ACCF/AHA Guideline Recommendations): a report of the American College of Cardiology Foundation/American Heart Association Task Force on Practice Guidelines. J Am Coll Cardiol 61:1555–1570

20. Li Q, Zeng H, Liu F, Shen J, Li L, Zhao J et al (2015) High Ankle-Brachial Index Indicates Cardiovascular and Peripheral Arterial Disease in Patients With Type 2 Diabetes. Angiology. doi:10.1177/0003319715573657

21. de Liefde II, Hoeks SE, van Gestel YR, Klein J, Bax JJ, Verhagen HJ et al (2009) The prognostic value of impaired walking distance on long-term outcome in patients with known or suspected peripheral arterial disease. Eur J Vasc Endovasc Surg 38:482–487

22. American Diabetes Association (2014) Standards of medical care in diabetes – 2014. Diabetes Care 37(Suppl 1):S14–S80

23. Conen D, Everett BM, Kurth T, Creager MA, Buring JE, Ridker PM et al (2011) Smoking, smoking cessation, [corrected] and risk for symptomatic peripheral artery disease in women: a cohort study. Ann Intern Med 154:719–726

24. Phillips SA, Mahmoud AM, Brown MD, Haus JM (2014) Exercise interventions and peripheral arterial function: implications for cardio-metabolic disease. Prog Cardiovasc Dis. doi:10.1016/j.pcad.2014.12.005

25. Fokkenrood HJ, Lauret GJ, Verhofstad N, Bendermacher BL, Scheltinga MR, Teijink JA (2015) The effect of supervised exercise therapy on

physical activity and ambulatory activities in patients with intermittent claudication. Eur J Vasc Endovasc Surg 49:184–191

26. Ashworth NL, Chad KE, Harrison EL, Reeder BA, Marshall SC (2005) Home versus center based physical activity programs in older adults. Cochrane Database Syst Rev. doi:10.1002/14651858.CD004017. pub2CD004017

27. Gardner AW, Poehlman ET (1995) Exercise rehabilitation programs for the treatment of claudication pain. A meta-analysis. JAMA 274:975–980

28. Gaede P, Lund-Andersen H, Parving HH, Pedersen O (2008) Effect of a multifactorial intervention on mortality in type 2 diabetes. N Engl J Med 358:580–591

29. Mondillo S, Ballo P, Barbati R, Guerrini F, Ammaturo T, Agricola E et al (2003) Effects of simvastatin on walking performance and symptoms of intermittent claudication in hypercholesterolemic patients with peripheral vascular disease. Am J Med 114:359–364

30. Mohler ER 3rd, Hiatt WR, Creager MA (2003) Cholesterol reduction with atorvastatin improves walking distance in patients with peripheral arterial disease. Circulation 108:1481–1486

31. Mehler PS, Coll JR, Estacio R, Esler A, Schrier RW, Hiatt WR (2003) Intensive blood pressure control reduces the risk of cardiovascular events in patients with peripheral arterial disease and type 2 diabetes. Circulation 107:753–756

32. Mancia G, Fagard R, Narkiewicz K, Redon J, Zanchetti A, Bohm M et al (2014) 2013 ESH/ESC Practice guidelines for the management of arterial hypertension. Blood Press 23:3–16

33. Fowkes FG, Price JF, Stewart MC, Butcher I, Leng GC, Pell AC et al (2010) Aspirin for prevention of cardiovascular events in a general population screened for a low ankle brachial index: a randomized controlled trial. JAMA 303:841–848

34. Berger JS, Krantz MJ, Kittelson JM, Hiatt WR (2009) Aspirin for the prevention of cardiovascular events in patients with peripheral artery disease: a meta-analysis of randomized trials. JAMA 301:1909–1919

35. Baigent C, Blackwell L, Collins R, Emberson J, Godwin J, Peto R et al (2009) Aspirin in the primary and secondary prevention of vascular disease: collaborative meta-analysis of individual participant data from randomised trials. Lancet 373:1849–1860

36. Pande RL, Hiatt WR, Zhang P, Hittel N, Creager MA (2010) A pooled analysis of the durability and predictors of treatment response of cilostazol in patients with intermittent claudication. Vasc Med 15:181–188

37. Goodney PP, Beck AW, Nagle J, Welch HG, Zwolak RM (2009) National trends in lower extremity bypass surgery, endovascular interventions, and major amputations. J Vasc Surg 50:54–60

38. Slovut DP, Lipsitz EC (2012) Surgical technique and peripheral artery disease. Circulation 126:1127–1138